T0176951

**Emergency Care
and the Public's Health**

# Emergency Care and the Public's Health

Edited by

**Jesse M. Pines,** MD, MBA, MSCE
Director, Office for Clinical Practice Innovation
Professor of Emergency Medicine and Health Policy
The George Washington University
Washington, DC, USA

**Jameel Abualenain,** MD, MPH
Assistant Professor of Emergency Medicine
Department of Emergency Medicine
The George Washington University
Washington, DC, USA;
King Abdulaziz University
Jeddah, Saudi Arabia

**James Scott,** MD
Professor of Emergency Medicine and Health Policy
The George Washington University School of Medicine and Health Science
Washington, DC, USA

**Robert Shesser,** MD, MPH
Professor and Chair
Department of Emergency Medicine
The George Washington University
Washington, DC, USA

WILEY Blackwell

This edition first published 2014 © 2014 by John Wiley & Sons Ltd

*Registered office:* John Wiley & Sons, Ltd, The Atrium, Southern Gate, Chichester, West Sussex, PO19 8SQ, UK

*Editorial offices:* 9600 Garsington Road, Oxford, OX4 2DQ, UK
The Atrium, Southern Gate, Chichester, West Sussex, PO19 8SQ, UK
111 River Street, Hoboken, NJ 07030-5774, USA

For details of our global editorial offices, for customer services and for information about how to apply for permission to reuse the copyright material in this book please see our website at www.wiley.com/wiley-blackwell

The right of the authors to be identified as the authors of this work has been asserted in accordance with the UK Copyright, Designs and Patents Act 1988.

*Library of Congress Cataloging-in-Publication Data*

Emergency care and the public's health / edited by Jesse M. Pines, Jameel Abualenain, James Scott, Robert Shesser.
    p. ; cm.
Includes bibliographical references and index.
ISBN 978-1-118-77980-4 (cloth)
I. Pines, Jesse M., editor of compilation. II. Abualenain, Jameel, 1980- editor of compilation.
III. Scott, James L., editor of compilation. IV. Shesser, Robert, editor of compilation.
[DNLM: 1. Emergency Service, Hospital–organization & administration–United States. 2. Public Health Practice–United States. WX 215]
RA645.5
362.18068–dc23
                                            2014000618

A catalogue record for this book is available from the British Library.

Wiley also publishes its books in a variety of electronic formats. Some content that appears in print may not be available in electronic books.

Cover image: iStockphoto.com #15760827 © 2011 4X-image and iStockphoto.com #16755915 © 2011 svedoliver
Cover design by Modern Alchemy

Typeset in 10/13pt Palatino by Laserwords Private Limited, Chennai, India
Printed and bound in Malaysia by Vivar Printing Sdn Bhd

1   2014

# Contents

Editor Biographies, vii

List of Contributors, xi

Foreword, xv

## Part 1 The US emergency care system

**1** The emergency care system in the United States, 3
*Jesse M. Pines and Jameel Abualenain*

**2** Ten common misconceptions about emergency care, 11
*Dana R. Sax and Robert Shesser*

**3** International perspectives on emergency care, 21
*Jameel Abualenain, Drew Richardson, David Mountain, Samuel Vaillancourt, Michael Schull, Phillip Anderson, Eric Revue, Brijal Patel, Ali Pourmand, Hamid Shokoohi, Shingo Hori, Lit-Sin Quek, and Suzanne Mason*

## Part 2 Technology in emergency care

**4** Human factors in emergency care, 47
*Raj M. Ratwani, A. Zach Hettinger, and Rollin J. Fairbanks*

**5** Information technology in emergency care, 59
*Adam Landman and E. Gregory Marchand*

**6** Telehealth and acute care, 75
*Sara Paradise, Michael Kee-Ming Shu, and Neal Sikka*

**7** Simulation in emergency care, 87
*Claudia Ranniger and Keith E. Littlewood*


**Part 3 Emergency care workforce**

**8** Emergency care workforce projections, 99
*James Scott, Rachelle Pierre-Mathew, and Drew Maurano*


**Part 4 Emergency preparedness and response
to emergencies and disasters**

**9** US emergency and disaster response in the past, present, and
future: The multi-faceted role of emergency health care, 113
*Joseph A. Barbera and Anthony G. Macintyre*

**10** Emergency public health, 127
*Rebecca Katz, Anthony Macintyre, and Joseph Barbera*


**Part 5 Emergency care payment reform and legal issues**

**11** The role of the emergency department in care coordination, 141
*Emily R. Carrier*

**12** Payment reform in emergency care, 151
*Janice Blanchard, Stephanie Donald, and Nathan Seth Trueger*

**13** The legal framework for hospital emergency care, 169
*Sara Rosenbaum*

**14** The future of emergency medicine, 191
*Robert Shesser*

Index, 201

# Editor Biographies

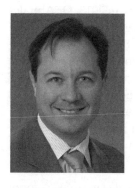 **Jesse M. Pines**, MD, MBA, MSCE is the Director of the Office for Clinical Practice Innovation and a Professor of Emergency Medicine and Health Policy at The George Washington University. He is also a board-certified emergency physician. Dr Pines has served as a Senior Advisor to the Center for Medicare and Medicaid Innovation at the Center for Medicare and Medicaid Services in the US government, and has consulted for the National Quality Forum and the Institute of Medicine. Dr Pines holds a Bachelor of Arts and a Master of Science in Clinical Epidemiology from the University of Pennsylvania as well as a Medical Degree and a Master of Business Administration from Georgetown University. He completed a residency in emergency medicine at the University of Virginia and a fellowship in research at the Center for Clinical Epidemiology and Biostatistics at the University of Pennsylvania. He has received grant funding from several government agencies and private foundations to conduct research and is author of over 170 peer-reviewed publications. He has authored two other Wiley books: *Evidence Based Emergency Care: Diagnostic Testing and Clinical Decision Rules*, 2nd edition (2013), and *Visual Diagnosis in Emergency and Critical Care Medicine*, 2nd edition (2011). He lives in Fairfax, VA with his wife Lori, and three children, Asher, Molly, and Oren.

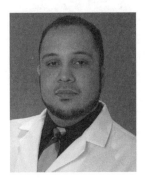

**Jameel Abualenain**, MD MPH is an Assistant Professor of Emergency Medicine at the George Washington University. He is a board-certified emergency physician and works as an attending physician at the George Washington University Hospital. He is also a faculty member in the Department of Emergency Medicinea at King Abdulaziz University, Jeddah, Saudi Arabia. He received an MBBS (MD) degree from King Abdulaziz University, Jeddah, Saudi Arabia in 2004 as well as a Master of Public Health in Management from the George Washington University in 2013. Dr Abualenain completed his internship and residency in emergency medicine at the George Washington University in 2011 and received the Excellence in Resident Research Award. He completed a two-year fellowship in Emergency Care Operations and Health Policy in 2013 and currently completing a one-year fellowship in Simulation and Medical Education, as well as Master Teacher, Leadership, and Development graduate certificate at the George Washington University. He has co-authored many peer-reviewed publications and has presented at emergency medicine conferences nationally.

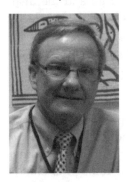

**James Scott**, MD, served as Dean of the George Washington School of Medicine and Health Sciences (SMHS) from July 2003 through December 2010. Previously, he served as residency director, Associate Dean for Graduate Medical Education, and Assistant Dean for Student Affairs in SMHS. Since stepping down as dean, Dr Scott has devoted his time and energy to improving medical education in Africa. He is Co-Principal Investigator on the Medical Education Partnership Initiative, a $130 million grant from the NIH and HRSA to improve the quantity, quality and retention of doctors in sub-Saharan Africa. He also serves as senior academic adviser to the Global Health Service Partnership, a program through the Peace Corps places American medical educators in African medical schools. In addition to publishing many academic articles and chapters, he has been the recipient of several teaching awards both at the George Washington University and nationally. Dr Scott received his bachelor's degree from the University of Notre Dame in 1977 followed by serving in the Peace Corps in Sierra Leone, West Africa. He received his medical degree from the University of Arizona College of Medicine in 1983. Dr Scott completed his internal medicine internship at the University of Arizona and did his emergency medicine residency at the George Washington University.

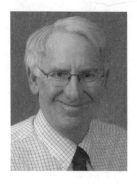

**Robert Shesser**, MD, MPH is currently Chair of the Department of Emergency Medicine at the George Washington University and is a tenured Professor of Emergency Medicine, Medicine, and International Health. He received a BA degree from the University of Rochester in 1971, an MD degree from the University of Miami in 1976 and an MPH from Johns Hopkins University in 1987. He completed an internal medicine residency at the George Washington University Hospital in 1979 and is a Diplomate of the American Board of Internal Medicine and American Board of Emergency Medicine.

During his career at the George Washington University, since joining the faculty in 1979 Dr Shesser has held numerous leadership positions including Interim Chief Executive Officer of the Medical Faculty Associates, 1996–1998, Associate Medical Director of the George Washington Health Plan 1999–2000, Vice Chair of the Department of Emergency Medicine 1985–1995, and Director of the Emergency Medicine Residency Program 1985–1995.

He is currently responsible for managing the physician practice of three emergency departments: the George Washington University Hospital ED (75 000 patient visits per year), the Walter Reed National Medical Center, and the Washington VA Hospital.

Academic achievements include management of a number of government and private sector grants in injury epidemiology and control, international emergency medicine development, and general clinical care. He has lectured or consulted internationally in Italy, Egypt, Hungary, Romania, Iceland, Estonia, Chile, and Saudi Arabia. Dr Shesser has published numerous papers in peer-reviewed journals on general clinical topics, emergency medicine education, and emergency medicine administration, and has spoken both domestically and internationally on a variety of administrative and clinical topics.

# List of Contributors

**Jameel Abualenain, MD, MPH**
Assistant Professor of Emergency Medicine
The George Washington University
Washington, DC, USA;
King Abdulaziz University
Jeddah, Saudi Arabia

**Phillip Anderson, MD**
Assistant Professor, Harvard Medical School
Department of Emergency Medicine, Beth
Israel Deaconess Medical Center
Boston, MA, USA

**Joseph A. Barbera, MD**
Associate Professor of Engineering
Management (Crisis and Emergency
Management)
Clinical Associate Professor of Emergency
Medicine
Co-Director, Institute for Crisis, Disaster, and
Risk Management
Department of Engineering Management and
Systems Engineering
The George Washington University
Washington, DC, USA

**Janice Blanchard, MD, MPH, PhD**
Associate Professor of Emergency Medicine
Chief, Health Policy Section, Department of
Emergency Medicine
The George Washington University
Washington, DC, USA

**Emily R. Carrier, MD, MSc**
Senior Health Researcher
Center for Studying Health System Change
Washington, DC, USA

**Stephanie Donald, MD**
Health Policy Fellow Health Policy Fellow
Adjunct Instructor of Emergency Medicine
The George Washington University
Washington, DC, USA

**Rollin J. Fairbanks, MD, MS**
Director, National Center for Human Factors in
Healthcare, MedStar Institute for Innovation
Associate Professor of Emergency Medicine,
Georgetown University School of Medicine
Washington, DC, USA;
Adjunct Associate Professor of Industrial
Systems Engineering, University at Buffalo
Buffalo, NY, USA

**Zach Hettinger, MD, MS**
Assistant Professor of Emergency Medicine
Director of Informatics Research
Georgetown University School of Medicine
National Center for Human Factors in
Healthcare
Washington, DC, USA

**Shingo Hori, MD**
Professor and Chairman
Emergency and Critical Care Medicine
Keio University, School of Medicine
Tokyo, Japan

**Rebecca Katz, PhD, MPH**
Associate Professor
Department of Health Policy
The George Washington University,
School of Public Health and
Health Services
Washington, DC, USA

**Adam Landman, MD, MS, MIS, MHS**
Chief Medical Information Officer for Health
Information Innovation and Integration
Brigham and Women's Hospital
Boston, MA;
Associate Physician, Department of
Emergency Medicine
Assistant Professor, Harvard Medical School
Boston, MA, USA

**Keith E. Littlewood, MD**
Assistant Dean
School of Medicine
University of Virginia
Charlottesville, VA, USA

**Anthony MacIntyre, MD**
Professor of Emergency Medicine
The George Washington University
Washington, DC, USA

**E. Gregory Marchand, MD**
Director of Informatics, Department of
Emergency Medicine
MedStar Washington Hospital Center
Associate Medical Director
MedSTAR Transport Services
Washington, DC, USA

**Suzanne Mason, MBBS, FRCS, MD,
FCEM**
Professor of Emergency Medicine
EMRiS group
School of Health and Related Research
University of Sheffield
Sheffield, UK

**Drew Maurano, PA-C**
Associate Clinical Professor
Director, Event Medicine
Department of Emergency Medicine
The George Washington University
Washington, DC, USA

**David Mountain, MBBS, FACEM**
Associate professor, Head of Department
Emergency Medicine
University of Western Australia
Academic Emergency Medicine/ Sir Charles
Gairdner Hospital Emergency Department
Perth, Western Australia, Australia

**Sara Paradise, BA, MD Candidate**
The George Washington University
Washington, DC, USA

**Brijal Patel, MD MPH**
Emergency Physician
Department of Emergency Medicine
The George Washington University
Washington, DC, USA

**Rachelle Pierre-Mathew, MD, MPP**
Assistant Professor of Emergency
Medicine
The George Washington University
Washington, DC, USA

**Jesse M. Pines, MD, MBA, MSCE**
Director, Office for Clinical Practice
Innovation
Professor of Emergency Medicine and Health
Policy
The George Washington University
Washington, DC, USA

**Ali Pourmand, MD, MPH, RDMS**
Assistant Professor of Emergency Medicine
Director, Educational Technology, Department
of Emergency Medicine
The George Washington University
Washington, DC, USA

**Lit-Sin Quek, MBBS, MRCS Ed, MMed**
Head of Department and Senior Consultant
Alexandra Hospital, Junghealth Services
Singapore

**Claudia Ranniger, MD, PhD**
Assistant Professor of Emergency Medicine
Director of Simulation, The Clinical Learning
and Simulation Skills Center
Office of Interdisciplinary Medicine and the
Department of Emergency Medicine
The George Washington University
Washington, DC, USA

**Raj Ratwani, PhD**
Scientific Director
National Center for Human Factors in
Healthcare
MedStar Institute for Innovation MedStar
Health Research Institute
Washington, DC, USA

**Eric Revue, MD**
Emergency Physician Toxicologist
Head of the Emergency Department and
Prehospital EMS (SMUR) Louis Pasteur
Hospital
Chartres (France) French Society of EM
Chair of the website of the EuSEM (European
Society of EM)

**Drew Richardson, MBBS, FACEM,
GradCertHE**
Associate Professor
Emergency Department, Australian National
University Medical School
Canberra, Australia

**Sara Rosenbaum, JD**
Harold and Jane Hirsh Professor
Department of Health Policy
The George Washington
University, School of Public Health and Health
Services
Washington, DC, USA

**Dana R. Sax, MD, MPH**
Emergency Physician
Kaiser East Bay Medical Center
Oakland, CA, USA

**Michael J. Schull, MD, MSc, FRCPC**
CEO and President, Institute for Clinical
Evaluative Sciences; CIHR Applied Chair in
Health
Services and Policy Research;
Professor, Department of Medicine, University
of Toronto; Staff Physician, Emergency
Department, Sunnybrook Health Sciences
Centre
Sunnybrook Health Sciences Centre and
Institute for Clinical Evaluative Sciences (ICES)
Toronto, ON, Canada

**James Scott, MD**
Professor of Emergency Medicine and Health
Policy

The George Washington University School of
Medicine and Health Science
Washington, DC, USA

**Robert Shesser, MD, MPH**
Professor and Chair
Department of Emergency Medicine
The George Washington University
Washington, DC, USA

**Hamid Shokoohi, MD, MPH, RDMS**
Assistant Professor of Emergency Medicine
Director, Emergency Ultrasound Fellowship,
Department of Emergency Medicine
The George Washington University
Washington, DC, USA

**Michael Kee-Ming Shu, BS, MD
Candidate**
The George Washington University
Washington, DC, USA

**Neal Sikka, MD**
Associate Professor of Emergency
Medicine
Director Innovative Practice and Telehealth
Section, Department of Emergency
Medicine
The George Washington University
Washington, DC, USA

**Nathan Seth Trueger, MD**
Health Policy Fellow, Adjunct Instructor of
Emergency Medicine
Department of Emergency Medicine
The George Washington University
Washington, DC, USA

**Samuel Vaillancourt, MD CM, MPH,
FRCP(C)**
Clinical Associate and Health Policy Research
Fellow
Emergency Department and Li Ka Shing
Knowledge Institute, St. Michael's Hospital
Toronto, ON, Canada

# Foreword

The Flexner Report, published in 1910 with the support of the Carnegie Foundation, literally transformed the face of American medicine. Flexner called on American medical schools to enact higher admission and education standards and embrace mainstream science in its teaching and research. Medical schools responded, and modern approach to medicine was born.

Today, Abraham Flexner's influence is still strong. In fact, US medical education has not changed much from the framework Flexner proposed more than 100 years ago. All that has changed is the world in which modern doctors, including emergency physicians, practice.

If the twentieth century was about science, the twenty-first century is about systems. The scientific basis of health care is as important as ever, but it has grown more complex and interconnected than Flexner could have imagined in 1910. We not only know far more about the molecular mechanisms of health and disease, but we also know vastly more about the influence of social and behavioral science, environmental health, nutrition, early life experiences, family dynamics, human factors engineering, health literacy, operations science, information technology, team-based care, and numerous other considerations.

There are few domains in modern medicine where reliance on systems is more necessary than in emergency care. Emphatically, emergency medicine is a team sport. Although the specialty is barely more than 50 years old, it has evolved dramatically from the days when its practitioners learned on the job, or a few years later, rotated for a month or two on every other clinical service in the hospital. Today, emergency medicine is a dynamic and growing specialty that is not only adept at providing life-saving care, but also performs advanced diagnostic workups, delivers urgent care, manages disasters and other threats to population health, oversees delivery of emergency medicine services, provides efficient after-hours acute care, and serves as the "safety net of the safety net" for the poor and the uninsured.

On any shift, an emergency physician may interact with over a hundred professional colleagues and an even larger number of patients and family members speaking a wide array of languages. In addition to being adept at physical diagnosis and clinical procedures; a modern emergency physician must be comfortable with health information technology, crew resource management, collaborative practice, patient engagement, global health, telemedicine, disaster preparedness, and other considerations. If not, he or she will be unable to practice in an efficient, effective, and compassionate way.

Current textbooks on emergency medicine are not adapted to this brave new world. Most are grounded in the Flexnerian tradition, and are designed to cover one disease at a time. This book is different. It offers readers a comprehensive look at our modern emergency care system, and examines how it can contribute to public health.

Knowledge of systems is essential to the modern practice of emergency medicine. It is no longer enough to be able to make order out of chaos at the bedside. That is still important, but a modern emergency physician must also know how to make order out of chaos in a still too fragmented delivery system, and do so in ways that promote patient safety, clinical efficiency, and the health of the community.

Read, learn, and enjoy.

**Arthur L. Kellermann, MD, MPH**
Dean, F. Edward Hébert School of Medicine
Uniformed Services University of the Health Sciences

PART 1

# The US emergency care system

CHAPTER 1

# The emergency care system in the United States

**Jesse M. Pines[1] and Jameel Abualenain[1,2]**

[1]*Emergency Medicine and Health Policy, The George Washington University, USA*
[2]*King Abdulaziz University, Saudi Arabia*

## Introduction

Over the past 4–5 decades, care in hospital-based emergency departments (EDs) has undergone a fundamental transformation. Emergency care of the 1960s and 1970s in the United States was delivered in the "emergency room" or "ER": literally, a small location or room within the hospital where a limited number of after-hours emergencies were seen. Then, the rest of the hospital was basically closed. ERs of the past had no legislative requirement to see patients who could not pay, and providers who worked there were not formally trained in emergency care.

Fast forward to 2013 and the large EDs of today are very different: sprawling departments with 50–100 separate patient rooms, immediate access to advanced technology, highly trained staff, and a federal mandate that all patients require medical screening examinations regardless of their ability to pay. The twenty-first century ED serves as the staging area for the critically ill and injured, an always-open location that provides high-quality acute unscheduled care, and has a critical role in the nation's safety net. While the ERs of the past arguably played a small part in the public's health, the ED of today plays a critical one, and the role seems to expand year after year. EDs are increasingly the "front door" of the hospital, currently the source of approximately half of inpatient admissions to US hospitals.[1] EDs are the critical pivot point where patients from all walks of life have life-threatening diseases excluded or receive prompt treatment.

*Emergency Care and The Public's Health*, First Edition.
Edited by Jesse M. Pines, Jameel Abualenain, James Scott and Robert Shesser.
© 2014 John Wiley & Sons, Ltd. Published 2014 by John Wiley & Sons, Ltd.

Today's US EDs have tremendous diagnostic therapeutic tools, resources (such as computed tomography (CT), ultrasound, and laboratory testing), and expertise at their disposal to deliver high-quality care. Yet, EDs simultaneously suffer from the wider systemic problems in the US health care system.

• ED care is highly fragmented. Often, ED providers have little knowledge of patients' medical history beyond what patients can recount, or what information resides in their local hospital records. It is not uncommon that patients' primary care providers (PCPs) never receive the clinical information of an ED encounter.

• The past decade has seen dramatic increases in the use of diagnostic technology in the ED, namely CT scans and laboratory testing. A recent study found that the number of CTs grew 330% from 3.2% in 1996 to 13.9% in 2007.[2] While the CT has been transformational in the practice of emergency care, dramatic increases also mean there may be overuse. This is a particular issue in trauma patients, and in some trauma centers the CT seems to have replaced a careful physical examination.

• ED crowding is a major problem that exists in more than 9 out of 10 US hospitals. ED care delivered during these more crowded periods has been associated with several negative clinical outcomes including poorer patient satisfaction, higher rates of complications and mortality, and lower quality of care.[3] Several solutions exist that can improve crowding, and in some cases eliminate it, yet these interventions are underused.[4]

• Electronic health records (EHRs) – which are now being woven into the fabric of US hospitals – solve many problems such as doctors' poor handwriting. Yet, at the same time, many EHRs are often difficult to use and can dramatically hinder ED performance during their implementation. Some create systematic errors, and most systems are not interoperable: information kept in one system cannot be shared with other systems easily.[5]

The objective of *Emergency Care and The Public's Health* is to offer readers a guided tour through the history and current state of America's EDs, with a glimpse into emergency care systems from other parts of the world. This book describes the successes of emergency care, and also provides an honest appraisal of what can be improved.

This book started as a collaboration among ED physicians, the Health Policy, Engineering, and Law faculties at the George Washington University in Washington, DC, who came together in 2011–2012 to present a University Seminar Series aimed at exploring the major issues in emergency care and public health. The book is the result of that Seminar Series; it is not intended to be comprehensive, but rather a primer for emergency care providers, researchers, policymakers, and other interested stakeholders into the details of what really happens every day in EDs, and how it can be improved.

## A journey through the myths and misconceptions of emergency care

Before launching into any discussion about emergency care, it is first vital to dispel common myths and misconceptions about the ED. Ask an average American about ED care and conventional wisdom is that EDs are overrun primarily with the uninsured, homeless, and immigrant populations, who mostly use EDs for unnecessary "inappropriate" reasons. In reality, a low proportion of ED care is for low-acuity illness, and the demographics of the ED resembles the insurance makeup of the country and local community. Most patients seen in the ED, in fact, have private health insurance. The problem is that many of the EDs portrayed on TV tend to be in poorer socioeconomically disadvantaged areas.

For example, *The Waiting Room* (2012), a documentary that depicted the triumphs and sorrows of ED care at Highland General Hospital in Oakland, California, focused on care for the disadvantaged, uninsured, and downtrodden. The movie was compelling, but nevertheless propagated the myth that EDs are about poor people. In fact, America's EDs are about everyone: the insurance mix of an ED tends to reflect the insurance mix of the community that surrounds the hospital, which can give false impressions about who actually uses the ED.

Myths about frequent users are also common. People think that those who repeatedly use the ED do not have their own doctors. In reality, frequent users of ED care are frequent users of overall health care, including PCPs.

Several other misconceptions abound, such as the ability to determine the "appropriateness" of ED care, who needs to be in the hospital, and whether there is robust quality measurement for most care delivered in the ED.

## A look at international emergency care

While it may be difficult to change how the average American sees the ED, one lens to change perspectives is to explore care delivered outside the United States. Some emergency care systems resemble that in the the United States, such as Australia, New Zealand, Canada, and the United Kingdom, where EDs are organized within hospitals. Yet, in those countries, there is a much greater focus on ensuring – in fact requiring – patients to move in and out quickly. France has a much greater emphasis on treating ambulance patients in the field, where anesthesiologists and nurse anesthetists commonly staff ambulances and can treat and release patients outside of the hospital setting. Less developed countries, such as Iran and India, have plans in place to enhance the workforce and emergency care capacities across the pre-hospital and ED systems. The common theme across many countries is continued development of emergency care systems, including enhancements in pre-hospital services, expanding the capacities of EDs, and improvements in the workforce where more highly trained staff are available in EDs to treat broadly heterogeneous conditions.

## First generation ED electronic health records 1.0

A major change in the past decade in the United States has been the proliferation of EHRs. EHRs are designed to manage patient data and records. The idea is that instead of combing through mountains of paper, providers can retrieve up-to-date records about patients with a simple keystroke. Medication errors – such as a patient receiving magnesium in place of morphine because of illegible scrawl by the doctor – would be eliminated. But the history of EHRs in the ED is not a simple one, and is rapidly evolving. While EHRs have solved some problems, they create others. Circa 2013, hospitals have rapidly installed EHRs from various vendors, who viciously compete for market share with one another, yet have not figured out ways in which systems can share data easily. How issues of interoperability and usability get resolved in the marketplace and by government regulation will determine whether EHRs in the ED are a net benefit or just a time-consuming distraction that takes providers away from the bedside.

## The human factor in emergency care

Conceptualizing the benefits and potential problems of EHRs is about understanding how human beings interact with their environments. EDs and ED care is extraordinarily complex: ED providers are required to manage multiple complex tasks simultaneously, but are frequently interrupted. Medical errors are a major problem in US hospitals, and EDs are no exception. The question is how researchers can identify and overcome these problems. Human factors engineering focuses on understanding the capabilities of the human user – the ED provider – and applies this knowledge to improve the tools they use (such as devices), machines, and systems (such as EHRs) with which the user and provider interact. The goal is to enhance the safety and efficiency of the process of providing care in the ED and understanding human factors is an important step to achieving that goal.

## Evolving technology: Telehealth and simulation

Two areas where technology has become increasingly important and will likely grow dramatically in the next decade in the ED are telehealth and simulation. Telehealth comes in multiple flavors, such as telemedicine, where real-time remote diagnostic services are changing the care of stroke patients. In some communities, tele-medicine provides rural hospitals with access to expert specialists, such as neurologists, to help them decide which stroke patients require thrombolytic therapy. Other technologies are evolving, such as store and forward technology, where clinicians can view data or images remotely to make recommendations. The major benefit of these remote technologies is that they provide critical access. Finally, mobile health or "mHealth," which uses smart phones, will likely become much more important in emergency care in the future, particularly in keeping track of patients after they leave the ED, transmitting health information, and gathering survey data. Simulation is vitally important because on-the-job training cannot adequately prepare ED providers for the variety of clinical presentations they are expected to manage. Simulation – and practice – is necessary to ensure providers are able to perform rare emergency procedures safely (e.g., cricothyroidotomy), appropriately evaluate complex presentations requiring coordination of multiple providers, and make decisions in resource-limited situations such as mass casualty events.

## What the future holds for the ED workforce

ED use has grown tremendously over the past few decades in the United States. Current expectations are that demands will continue to rise with an aging population, an increased focus on high technology medical care which is only available in the ED, and policy changes – such as the Affordable Care Act – which will result in millions more Americans with health insurance coverage. With current training programs in emergency medicine and projected retirements of emergency physicians, there is likely to be a shortage of trained emergency physicians for decades.

The shortage of emergency physicians will continue to expand the role of physician extenders – including physician assistants and nurse practitioners. In addition, new practice models for emergency care will need to be developed to meet these demands.

## Role of the ED in national preparedness

EDs and ED providers have been central in helping manage and mitigate the effects of disasters, and influencing how the nation responds to such events. The concept of emergency public health has emerged recently as a distinct discipline. Public health traditionally uses addresses population health issues and uses more traditional strategies such as using empirical research to drive policy change. Emergency public health has incorporated new methodologies and has emerged as a distinct discipline. Certain common public health practices related to crisis communications, epidemiologic investigations, and biosurveillance are vitally important during an emergency. However, principles of emergency management and medical care that distinguish preparedness and response actions and for managing rapidly evolving, unusual emergency situations are also being adopted to address population health during disasters.

## Evolving role of the ED in care coordination

Care coordination is emerging as a major concept in new health reform efforts. The goal is to ensure that, "patients' needs and preferences for health services and information sharing across people, functions and sites are met over time."[6] Care delivered in EDs has traditionally been a series of isolated provider–patient interactions that involve little interaction with other providers or elements of the healthcare system. The result is fragmentation and a lower quality of care because information is often lost, tests are sometimes duplicated, and care within episodic settings like EDs may not fit well into the larger plan of care, particularly when end-of-life goals are not communicated or available to ED providers. With greater emphasis on value, care coordination in the ED will become much more important in the future; specifically, with how ED providers coordinate care with each other, with other hospital-based providers, and across communities. Improved care coordination will be created through the development and promulgation of new quality metrics that ensure communication and information transfer at important pivot points (e.g., an ED visit or hospitalization). There are several models of care coordination, primarily involving improved communication across providers, ensuring interoperability across EHRs, and taking a more longitudinal approach to emergency care, where patients are called back after their ED visit and unmet needs addressed.

## How new payment reform policies will impact emergency care

Care coordination will be a centerpiece of how ED care will fit within the future "accountable" world of care in the United States, specifically the role of ED providers in enhancing the value of care delivered. This has been a major focus of provisions of the 2010 Affordable Care Act, which seek to expand access to care by expanding insurance coverage, through expanding the role of quality measurement, and using new models to pay for care. When it comes to acute and emergency care, enhancing value has not been a major focus, specifically through the structure of the fee-for-service (FFS) payment system. In the future, as new payment models become more prevalent, such as accountable care organizations, bundled payments, and episode-based payments, there will be increasing pressure on emergency care providers to take a closer look at the value of care provided. Attention will likely be focused on several areas that serve as major costs drivers: the role of the ED in admissions, and re-admissions, the expanding use of observation care, and on indications for advanced radiography use in the ED, along with efforts to bolster care coordination efforts.

## Legal issues in emergency care

One of the most important health care statutes in the United States has direct application to the ED: the Emergency Medical Treatment and Labor Act (EMTALA). EMTALA was the product of a long evolution which started at the turn of the twentieth century when physicians operated under the "no duty of care" common law principle. However, by the 1950s, the courts and legislatures were increasingly rejecting this principle, especially when it came to ED care. This was a reflection of both the unique vulnerability of ED patients – with EDs being the place where the public turned for acute health care when there was no other option – and the increasing power of the hospital industry. Today, EMTALA's screening, stabilization, and transfer requirements are established in common law and state law precedents. However, EMTALA continues to be controversial as it is often referred to as the archetypal "unfunded mandate" and it continues to evolve and to involve legal challenges as technology has improved and standards for emergency care have changed over time.

## Charting a course for the future of emergency care in the United States

Over the past decades, emergency care has undergone revolutionary changes in its structure, staffing, quality, and expectations – both medical and legal. In this ever-changing environment, emergency care leaders must develop robust adaptive organizations that provide future emergency physicians with the clinical and practice skills required for twenty-first century medical practice. It is likely that the 2013 practice of emergency care looks considerably different from how care will look in future decades because of changing payment and clinical models of care. The success of emergency medicine, especially compared with other medical specialties, will depend on how current leaders position the field in this rapidly changing environment.

## References

1 Pines JM, Mutter RL, Zocchi MS. Variation in emergency department admission rates across the United States. Med Care Res Rev. 2013;70(2):218–31.
2 Kocher KE, Meurer WJ, Fazel R, Scott PA, Krumholz HM, Nallamothu BK. National trends in use of computed tomography in the emergency department. Ann Emerg Med. 2011;58(5):452–62.e3.
3 Bernstein SL, Aronsky D, Duseja R, Epstein S, Handel D, Hwang U, et al.; Society for Academic Emergency Medicine, Emergency Department Crowding Task Force. The effect of emergency department crowding on clinically oriented outcomes. Acad Emerg Med. 2009;16(1):1–10.
4 Rabin E, Kocher K, McClelland M, Pines J, Hwang U, Rathlev N, et al. Solutions to emergency department 'boarding' and crowding are underused and may need to be legislated. Health Aff (Millwood). 2012;31(8):1757–66.
5 Farley HL, Baumlin KM, Hamedani AG, Cheung DS, Edwards MR, Fuller DC, et al. Quality and safety implications of emergency department information systems. Ann Emerg Med. 2013;62(4);399–407.
6 National Quality Forum: National Voluntary Consensus Standards for Coordination of Care across Episodes of Care and Care Transitions. Available at: http://www.qualityforum.org/Projects/c-d/Care_Coordination_Endorsement_Maintenance/Care_Coordination_Endorsement_Maintenance.aspx (accessed 10 December 2013).

# CHAPTER 2

# Ten common misconceptions about emergency care

## Dana R. Sax[1] and Robert Shesser[2]

[1]Kaiser East Bay Medical Center, CA
[2]Department of Emergency Medicine, The George Washington University, USA

## Misconception 1: EDs are crowded because large numbers of medically indigent patients use EDs for "primary care"

Multiple factors cause emergency department (ED) crowding. The current rate of annual ED utilization in the United States is slightly above 400 visits per 1000 population, and has increased 15% during the past decade.[1] The Institute of Medicine's 2006 report "Hospital-Based Emergency Care: At the Breaking Point" cited several drivers of ED crowding including increased numbers of ED visits, a shortage of on-call specialists, and lengthy delays prior to admission ("boarding").[2] While the ED serves as a "safety net" for the underserved, high volumes of low-acuity visits are not a major contributor to ED crowding. A recent study found that increasing diagnostic and treatment intensity was strongly associated with worsening ED crowding and that low-acuity use exerted a minimal impact.[3] In addition, multiple studies have found that prolonged times between an emergency physician's admitting decision and patient transfer from the ED to an inpatient bed ("ED boarding") is a major factor causing crowding.[4,5] Boarding has several causes, including inefficiencies resulting in slow transitions of care, inadequate inpatient capacity (bed space), and inadequate inpatient nurse staffing.

Peak ED patient arrival in many hospitals occurs in the late morning through mid-evening. The decision to admit generally occurs about 2.5 hours after arrival in the ED, so inpatient bed demands from most EDs accelerate during the late morning and early afternoon. Many hospital

*Emergency Care and The Public's Health*, First Edition.
Edited by Jesse M. Pines, Jameel Abualenain, James Scott and Robert Shesser.
© 2014 John Wiley & Sons, Ltd. Published 2014 by John Wiley & Sons, Ltd.

discharges occur later in the day because of the intensity and complexity of arranging outpatient services required for older, often lower income, and chronically ill patients with multiple comorbidities. The delays in discharging this category of patient result in longer ED waits for patients who arrive earlier in the day. The gap between peak ED arrival/admission rates and the availability of inpatient beds leading to ED crowding can also be attributed to an under-appreciated social service mission of the acute-care hospital.

## Misconception 2: Most ED patients are uninsured

Most ED patients are insured. The ED insurance mix mirrors the insurance mix of the general population in the hospital's catchment area. In the United States as a whole, the majority of US citizens have private insurance.[6] Patients with private insurance account for 35% of ED visits, those with Medicaid 22%, and those with Medicare 20%. Only 18% of visits are made by uninsured patients.[7] However, there is wide variation in payer mix, depending upon the hospital's location, which can contribute to the myth that "ED patients are uninsured" as ED patients in socioeconomically disadvantaged neighborhoods tend to be uninsured or covered by Medicaid (the government insurance for the poor). It is more a reflection of the insurance mix in the local neighborhood than of the ED itself, as ED patients in affluent neighborhoods have high rates of private insurance, again reflecting the local population. However, the rate of ED visits by the uninsured (452 visits per 1000 uninsured persons) is higher than the rate among the insured (367 visits per 1000 insured persons).[7] In the future, as more patients gain insurance through provisions of the Affordable Care Act (ACA), it is likely that fewer patients in the ED will be uninsured, similarly reflecting the insurance mix of the nation.

It has also been alleged that undocumented immigrants contribute significantly to ED costs. Several studies have shown that undocumented immigrants are less likely to use EDs than other populations.[8,9] These studies have found that, contrary to popular perceptions, communities with high ED use have fewer numbers of uninsured, Hispanic, and noncitizen residents. Noncitizens have 17 fewer visits per 100 people than citizens.[9]

## Misconception 3: EDs are inherently expensive relative to alternative outpatient settings for many visit categories

EDs are expensive because they require significant staffing and capital investment to achieve the core mission to evaluate and stabilize all patients experiencing life and limb-threatening emergencies. ED-based care is estimated to represent 2–6% of the total yearly US health care expenditure of $2.4 trillion per year.[10–14]

Much of the confusion concerning the relative cost of an ED visit results from widespread misunderstandings about the definitions of hospital costs (the hospital's actual costs to care for an individual), hospital charges (the itemized bill that the individual receives), and prices (the amount the individual or their insurer actually pays). The fundamental issue is how the actual hospital costs are attributed to individual patient encounters. For example, a recent survey found that patients are charged up to 700% more for the same procedures at different institutions.[15]

The cost attribution problem applies ED charges because the intense, high technology care delivered to the critically ill and to patients requiring intensive lab work and cross-sectional imaging often leads to cost misallocation among different categories of ED patient. When a portion of the capital costs for computed tomography (CT) or magnetic resonance imaging (MRI) scanners are attributed to low-acuity ED patients, their bills are much higher than those that would be received in alternative outpatient settings. High intensity care is extraordinarily expensive, and probably not fully accounted for in bills received by critically ill patients.

Another way that investigators have approached the issue of ED costs has been to calculate marginal costs of treating a low-acuity ED patient. This approach recognizes that once capacity is installed to fulfill the ED's core mission(s), excess capacity can be leveraged to treat minor visits at little additional cost. As befits a confusing area, estimates of the marginal cost for a low-acuity ED visit vary from $24 to $300–400.[14,16] The true marginal cost of the lower acuity patients would likely be somewhere in the middle; more than an office visit, but not a societal "budget breaker" as is often claimed.

## Misconception 4: ED frequent users just use ED for their care and have no longitudinal care relationships with other doctors

Studies on "frequent fliers" have shown that heavy ED users tend to be high utilizers of health care in general, and often have multiple regular longitudinal relationships with a variety of physicians.[17,18] High ED users tend to be "sicker," have more comorbidities, and have complicated social situations requiring frequent use of a variety of treatment venues. For frequent users, ED physicians often spend considerable time coordinating outpatient treatment plan among multiple specialists caring for the patient. When such a patient requires admission, the emergency physician may have to devote much time to "negotiate" among different providers or services to which the patient can be admitted.

## Misconception 5: There are generally accepted guidelines about what constitutes "appropriate" ED use

The ED's optimal role in low-acuity ambulatory care has been fiercely debated.[19-23] The literature has frequently labeled utilization of the ED for low-acuity illness as "inappropriate." Decisions as to which visits on retrospective review are deemed "appropriate" depend on the criteria used and over 50 methods of categorizing visits as nonurgent have been identified in the literature.[22] Depending on the criteria used, the proportion of visits classified as nonurgent varies from 10% to 90%.[22,23] The wide variation suggests that the categorization methodologies lack reliability, accuracy, and reproducibility.

There is also an inherent value judgment when these visits are labeled "inappropriate." Reasons for using the ED are varied and based on individual patient situations and perceived need for care. A visit that is deemed "inappropriate" by an expert retrospective reviewer after a thorough workup leads to a benign diagnosis was probably deemed "potentially life-threatening" or certainly "urgent" by a patient with an alarming new symptom or acute pain. Patients choose the ED over other sites for many reasons including their perception of urgency, familiarity with the ED, lack of timely access to a regular provider, the ED's 24/7 open door policy where patients can be seen when and where they want regardless of their insurance, or because they have been referred there by another provider.

## Misconception 6: There are clear-cut guidelines about which ED patients should be admitted to the hospital

The percentage of total inpatient admissions originating in the ED has been steadily increasing in the United States. Over 50% of US inpatient admissions are now initiated in the ED, with an estimated mean per admission cost of $9200.[24] ED providers must make critical evaluation, treatment, and disposition decisions in a compressed time period, often with incomplete data, in a health care system that expects that no patient with a life-threatening illness is ever discharged home.

Although external case management guidelines such as Milliman & Robertson and Interqual are widely used by hospital case managers to stratify patients as "full" or "observation" admissions, these guidelines are, for the most part, based on expert opinion, and are infrequently used by ED physicians. Most admission decisions are made by an ED physician using subjective criteria without benefit of clear-cut guidelines or evidence-based criteria. The lack of provider-employed standardized admission guidelines results in wide variation in the percentage of ED patients who are admitted among different hospitals and among physicians within the same hospital.[24-26] This variation will be much lower for obvious high-acuity patients than for stable patients with symptoms such as syncope, generalized weakness, or nonfocal neurologic symptoms that could, but often do not represent subtle presentations of serious illness.

The subjective criteria used to make these decisions include the patient's clinical status, other comorbidities, preferences regarding admission, desires of their longitudinal care provider (or that provider's cross-coverage), social support situation including home or living situation, and the reliability of follow up. Community-acquired pneumonia is a good example of a condition where there are clear evidence-based admission criteria.[27] Yet, there is still substantial variation in admission decisions for pneumonia in the ED. Some of the variation can be attributed to local practice patterns, hospital or ED culture, or individual physician risk tolerance, and these factors can lead to significant differences in the efficiency of care. Admitting decisions may also be shaped by financial incentives as the fee-for-service system rewards admissions and more intensive resource utilization. Anecdotal reports abound concerning hospital administrators pressuring their ED groups to admit more patients.

## Misconception 7: Care for most conditions treated in the ED is carefully measured and reported to the public

There has been a strong recent push from private and government payers to develop and implement objective quality measurements in a variety of health care settings including the ED. These metrics are then disseminated to payers, the general public, and regulatory agencies who use the data for a variety of purposes.

The process of measure development is a lengthy one which involves a number of private and public organizations including the National Quality Forum, the Centers for Medicare and Medicaid Services (CMS), the Joint Commission, the Agency for Healthcare Research and Quality, and many specialty professional societies. A large number ED measures have been (or are about to be) implemented by CMS as part of its Hospital Compare Outpatient Quality Reporting initiative. The general categories in this program are: Timely and Effective Care; Readmissions, Complications and Deaths; Use of Medical Imaging; and a patient survey, Hospital Consumer Assessment of Healthcare Providers and Systems (HCAHPS).

Most ED-specific measures are currently in the Timely and Effective Care section. The measures that are largely under the control of ED physicians and staff include: door to ECG time for chest pain; door to balloon time for percutaneous intervention in patients with acute ST-segment elevation myocardial infarction; door to testing time for patients with acute stroke; blood cultures prior to antibiotics in patients with pneumonia; and appropriate antibiotic selection for those with community-acquired pneumonia. ED throughput measures that are reported include: door to discharge time for outpatients; door to admission time for inpatients; admission decision time to ED departure for inpatients; left without being seen rates; door to provider time; door to CT results reporting for "stroke symptom" patients; and door to analgesic time in patients with acute fractures.

The current ED measures are very much systemic in nature and are a blend of many subsystems that cut across a broad swathe of hospital operations. Their underlying premise seems to be that "faster is better," both for overall ED operations as well as time-dependent conditions such as myocardial infarction and stroke. However, there is a dearth of measures that can be used to assess the quality of care rendered by individual physicians. In the future, this will likely change as more measures are promulgated in the ED, particularly around the patient experience, and other various measures of disease-specific quality of care. Currently, aside from throughput measures, the quality of care for most ED patients is not systematically measured or reported.

Lack of quality data results in part because 70–80% of patients are discharged from the ED and follow-up data are generally unavailable or costly to obtain. Also, many ED patients have self-limited conditions that improve regardless of treatment, and the numbers of patients for whom evidence-based treatment measures can be applied is so small that years of data would be required to identify physicians whose care is substandard.

## Misconception 8: Emergency physicians are employed by the hospital and have a practice structure similar to other physicians at the hospital

Currently, the majority of ED physicians are contractors to the hospital. A 2011 survey determined that only 28% were employed by the hospital, with the remainder having a range of employment relationships with organizations that contract with the hospital for physician staffing of the ED.[28] This contracting model is also common in other hospital-based specialties (e.g. radiology, anesthesiology, pathology, critical care, and hospital medicine). In community hospitals, most other medical staff physicians have practices that are independent of hospital control. If the physician is in the position to "direct" admissions to different hospitals in a community, the physician is often treated as a "valued customer" by administrators of competing hospitals.

In order to maintain their ED contracts, independent emergency physician groups must provide service that is well accepted by both hospital administration and non-hospital-employed medical staff. This "service" often requires that the emergency group respond to a variety of clinical and administrative expectations from their medical staff colleagues. For the most part, this interaction occurs in a highly professional, collegial framework, but ongoing care must be exercised by the emergency group's leadership to maintain important medical staff alliances.

Contracted emergency medicine groups ultimately serve at the pleasure of the hospital's administration, not its medical staff. Standard contracts between the hospital and the ED group often include reciprocal "without cause" cancellation provisions. The trade press has cited many examples of disputes that arise from allegations that hospital administrations have terminated contracts of existing groups after receiving financial incentives to do so by the successor group. Although individual physicians are entitled to a hospital's medical staff "due process" protection, loss of the contract by the group that employs them may result in a requirement to resign from the medical staff.

The power imbalance between a hospital's administration and its ED physicians has been cited as a cause of increased resource utilization by emergency physicians whose ordering and admitting practices may be closely tracked by the hospital's administration. However, in most instances, physician and hospital incentives are aligned to provide prompt, patient-friendly, appropriate, and compassionate care. The current fee-for-service system permits the ED group to be independent of the hospital, because each party receives payments independent of the other. This may change in the future as new care models for the ED are developed under a payment system that rewards value over volume.

## Misconception 9: Most US acute care hospitals have the proper staff and equipment to care for all types of patient problems

Hospitals vary widely in the range of services they provide as a result of variations in the availability of both capital and human resources. An Institute of Medicine Report in 2007 found that only about 6% of EDs in the United States have all the supplies deemed essential for managing pediatric emergencies, and only half of hospitals have at least 85% of those supplies.[29] A 2003 survey by the American College of Emergency Physicians noted that about two-thirds of EDs across all regions of the United States documented inadequate on-call specialist coverage.[30] Of the 1427 hospitals that responded, 17% noted that some specialists had negotiated with their hospitals for fewer on-call coverage hours, 33% noted increased levels of transfers, and 37% were offering specialists incentives to be on call.[31]

Because health planning is organized at the state level, there is no standardized system for the definition of specialty centers and service regionalization throughout the United States. The most frequent regionalized services are adult trauma, pediatric trauma, and burn care. Recently, acute myocardial infarction and acute stroke centers have been developed. Hospitals that do not provide specific services have developed relationships with larger institutions for the rapid transfer of patients from the EDs of sending hospitals to their regional advanced care centers. Pre-hospital personnel in many jurisdictions make field triage decisions to take patients needing highly specialized services directly to the designated regional centers.

Many hospitals have experienced difficulty in providing certain services to ED patients that can be provided electively because of the reluctance of specialists to take ED calls. The provision of emergency specialist care to ED patients is driven by the perceived greater malpractice risk for the specialist than providing elective care to their regular patients, inconvenience, and the variable case mix where some patients are uninsured or have Medicaid insurance that pays very low rates. Hospitals have provided specialists with ED call stipends in an attempt to offset the opportunity costs of ED coverage. Nevertheless, the ED backup specialty coverage in many communities has a variety of coverage "holes" in its hospitals.

## Misconception 10: The ED workforce consists of physicians who failed to succeed in "private practice"

The modern specialty of EM began with physicians who had received general or specialty training in other disciplines, but were attracted to practicing in the ED and, over many years, evolved the specialty's boundaries and scope of practice. The first professional association, the American College of Emergency Physicians (ACEP) was formed in 1968, the first EM residency program (University of Cincinnati) was established in 1970, and the first EM board exam was administered in 1980.

The emergency care workforce evolved from practitioners who may not have explicitly chosen EM to a professionally committed and trained workforce for whom EM was their conscious career choice. Prior to the advent of trained EM specialists, many hospitals routinely staffed their ED with early career, non-EM specialists who were attempting to build their practices in the community by referring patients seen in the ED to themselves for aftercare.

The imbalance between patients' needs and EM workforce abilities provided the impetus for the growth of training programs. Between 1990 and 2002, the number of EM physicians in the United States increased by 79%, while the number of EM medical residents increased by 116%.[32] In 2009, there were 149 allopathic residency programs and 43 osteopathic EM residency programs.[33] In 2012, all 1668 offered positions for incoming EM residents were filled, and EM ranked fourth among all specialties chosen by US allopathic medical student seniors.[34] In 2007, only 35% of the EM workforce had not been "grandfathered" in from another training (i.e. had been practicing long enough to qualify for the EM boards) or were not trained in EM and board-certified. As the proportion of board-certified physicians continues to grow, and ED physicians advance in both academic and community settings, the "itinerant practitioner" myth will recede in the imaginations of both the medical profession and general public.

## References

1 Tang N, Stein J, Hsia RY, et al. Trends and characteristics of US emergency department visits, 1997–2007. J Am Med Assoc. 2010;304:664–70.
2 Institute of Medicine Committee on the Future of Emergency Care in the United States Health System. Hospital Based Emergency Care: At the Breaking Point. Washington, DC: National Academies Press, 2007.
3 Pitts SR, Pines JM, Handrigan MT, Kellermann AL. National trends in emergency department occupancy, 2001 to 2008: effect of inpatient admissions versus emergency department practice intensity. Ann Emerg Med. 2012;60(6):679–85.
4 Government Accountability Office. Hospital Emergency Departments: Crowded Conditions Vary Among Hospitals and Communities. GAO 03-460. 2003. Available at: http://www.gao.gov/new.items/d03460.pdf (accessed 26 November 2013).
5 Government Accountability Office. Hospital Emergency Departments: Crowding Continues to Occur, and Some Patients Wait Longer than Recommended Time Frames. GAO 09-347. 2009. Available at: http://www.gao.gov/assets/290/289048.pdf (accessed 26 November 2013).
6 Carlson JN, Menegazzi JJ, Callaway CW. Magnitude of national ED visits and resource utilization by the uninsured. Am J Emerg Med. 2013;31(4):722–6.
7 Owens PL, Mutter R. Payers of Emergency Department Care, 2006: Statistical Brief 77. Health care Cost and Utilization Project. Statistical Briefs. Rockville, MD: Agency for Health Care Policy and Research (US), 2006.
8 Cunningham P. What accounts for differences in the use of hospital emergency departments across US communities? Health Aff (Millwood). 2006;25(5):w324–36.
9 Derose KP, Bahney BW, Lurie N, Escarce JJ. Review: immigrants and health care access, quality and cost. Med Care Res Rev. 2009;66(4):335–08.
10 National Hospital Ambulatory Medical Care Survey. NHAMCS Micro-Data File, Centers for Disease Control and Prevention, 2010.
11 Pitts SR, Carrier ER, Rich EC, et al. Where Americans get acute care: increasingly it's not at their doctor's office. Health Aff (Millwood). 2010;29:91620–29.
12 Schuur JD, Venkatesh AK. The growing role of emergency departments in hospital admissions. New Engl J Med. 2012;367:391–3.
13 Lee MH, Schuur JD, Zink BJ. Owning the cost of emergency medicine: beyond 2%. Ann Emerg Med. 2013;62(5):498–505.
14 Williams RM. The costs of visits to emergency departments. New Engl J Med. 1996;334(10):642–6.
15 Medicare Provider Charge Data. Centers for Medicare and Medicaid Services. Available at: http://www.cms.gov/Research-Statistics-Data-and-Systems/Statistics-Trends-and-Reports/Medicare-Provider-Charge-Data/index.html (accessed 26 November 2013).
16 Bamezai A, Melnick G, Nawathe A. The cost of an emergency department visit and its relationship to emergency department volume. Ann Emerg Med. 2005;45(5):483–90.
17 Sun BC, Burstin HR, Brennan TA. Predictors and outcomes of frequent emergency department users. Acad Emerg Med. 2003;10(4):320–8.

18 LaCalle E, Rabin E. Frequent users of emergency departments: the myths, the data, and the policy implications. Ann Emerg Med. 2010;56(1):42–8.

19 Redstone P, Vancura JL, Barry D, Kutner JS. Nonurgent use of the emergency department. J Ambul Care Manage. 2008;31(4):370–6.

20 Afilalo J, Marinovich A, Afilalo M, Colacone A, Léger R, Unger B, et al. Nonurgent emergency department characteristics and barriers to primary care. Acad Emerg Med. 2004;11(12):1302–10.

21 Sempere-Selva T, Peiró S, Sendra-Pina P, Martínez-Espín C, López-Aguilera I. Inappropriate use of an accident and emergency department: magnitude, associated factors, and reasons – an approach with explicit criteria. Ann Emerg Med. 2001;37(6):568–79.

22 Durand AC, Gentile S, Devictor B, Palazzolo S, Vignally P, Gerbeaux P, et al. ED patients: how nonurgent are they? Systematic review of the emergency medicine literature. Am J Emerg Med. 2011;29(3):333–45.

23 Lowe RA, Bindman AB. Judging who needs emergency department care: a prerequisite for policy-making. Am J Emerg Med. 1997;15(2):133–6.

24 Morganti KG, Bauhoff S, Blanchard JC, Abir M, Iyer N, Smith A, et al. The Evolving Role of Emergency Departments in the United States. Rand Corporation. Available at: http://www.rand.org/pubs/research_reports/RR280 (accessed 26 November 2013).

25 Chen LM, Render M, Sales A, Kennedy EH, Wijtala W, Hofer TP. Intensive care unit admitting patterns in the Veterans Affairs health care system. Arch Intern Med. 2012;172(16):1220–6.

26 Studnicki J, Platanova EA, Fisher JW. Hospital-level variation in the percentage of admissions originating in the emergency department. Am J Emerg Med. 2012;30(8):1441–6.

27 Ewig S, de Roux A, Bauer T, García E, Mensa J, Niederman M, et al. Validation of prediction rules and indices for community acquired pneumonia. Thorax. 2004;59(5):421–7.

28 Medscape Physician Compensation Report: 2011. Available at: http://www.medscape.com/features/slideshow/compensation/2011/emergencymedicine (accessed 19 August 2013).

29 National Research Council. Emergency Care for Children: Growing Pains. Washington, DC: National Academies Press, 2007.

30 American College of Emergency Physicians (ACEP). On-call specialists coverage in US emergency departments. ACEP survey of emergency department directors: September 2004. Available at: www.acep.org/workarea/downloadasset.aspx?id=8974 (accessed 26 November 2013).

31 McConnell KJ, Johnson LA, Arab N, Richards CF, Newgard CD, Edlund T. The on-call crisis: a statewide assessment of the costs of providing on-call specialist coverage. Ann Emerg Med. 2007;49(6):727–33.

32 Perina DG, Collier RE, Thomas HA, et al. Report of the task force on residency training information (2007–2008), American Board of Emergency Medicine. Ann Emerg Med. 2008;51:671–9.

33 National Resident Matching Program, Results and Data: 2012 Main Residency Match.[SM] Washington, DC: National Resident Matching Program, 2012.

34 Counselman FL, Marco CA, Patrick VC, et al. A study of the workforce in emergency medicine: 2007. Am J Emerg Med. 2009;27:691–700.

# CHAPTER 3

# International perspectives on emergency care

Jameel Abualenain[1,2], Drew Richardson[3], David Mountain[4,5], Samuel Vaillancourt[6], Michael Schull[7,8,9], Phillip Anderson[10], Eric Revue[11], Brijal Patel[1], Ali Pourmand[1], Hamid Shokoohi[1], Shingo Hori[12], Lit-Sin Quek[13], and Suzanne Mason[14]

[1]Department of Emergency Medicine, The George Washington University, USA
[2]King Abdulaziz University, Saudi Arabia
[3]Emergency Department, Australian National University Medical School, Australia
[4]Department of Emergency Medicine, University of Western Australia, Australia
[5]Sir Charles Gairdner Hospital, Emergency Department, Australia
[6]Emergency Department and Li Ka Shing Knowledge Institute, Canada
[7]Department of Medicine, University of Toronto, Canada
[8]Emergency Department, Sunnybrook Health Sciences Centre, Institute for Clinical Evaluative Sciences (ICES), Canada
[9]Department of Emergency Services, Sunnybrook Health Sciences Centre, Canada
[10]Department of Emergency Medicine, Beth Israel Deaconess Medical Center, USA
[11]Emergency Department and Prehospital EMS (SMUR), France
[12]Emergency and Critical Care Medicine, Keio University, School of Medicine, Japan
[13]Alexandra Hospital, Juronghealth Services, Singapore
[14]EMR is group, School of Health and Related Research, University of Sheffield, UK

*Emergency Care and The Public's Health*, First Edition.
Edited by Jesse M. Pines, Jameel Abualenain, James Scott and Robert Shesser.
© 2014 John Wiley & Sons, Ltd. Published 2014 by John Wiley & Sons, Ltd.

## Introduction

This chapter describes emergency care systems across nine countries outside of the United States: Australia, Canada, Denmark, France, India, Iran, Japan, Singapore, and the United Kingdom. In each case, a local author, who is an emergency care leader in his country, provides some background and perspectives about their emergency care systems, how they are financed, crowding issues, and other challenges. Some of these countries have well-established emergency care systems with good infrastructure, workforce, and supportive societies. By comparison, many countries are still developing their systems. They face tremendous challenges and are struggling to fit emergency care in their health system. ED crowding is almost a universal theme in the included countries regardless of how well developed the country. Many of these countries established measures and interventions to reduce ED crowding with variable success and outcomes.

## Australia

Australia is an advanced, geographically large (approximately the size of the 48 contiguous US States), industrialized, and highly urbanized country (>85% urban), with a sparsely populated and vast outback. It is governed as a federal democracy comprised of six states and two territories. The main population centers are along the relatively fertile and irrigated southeast and southwest coastlines. In the outback, challenges include huge distances, poor access to advanced medical care, and relative economic disadvantage. Remote areas have high proportions of severely disadvantaged indigenous Australians, with very high rates of illness, both acute (e.g. infection and trauma) and chronic (e.g. rheumatic and ischemic heart disease, diabetes, and renal disease), and correspondingly very high usage of emergency services.

Most primary and specialist consultations occur in private "rooms," settings funded by federal government subsidies, patient payments, or health insurance (specialists only). Some supplemental services are directly funded or subsidized by governments, particularly where private practice is not viable. There is universal access to public hospitals and these institutions account for 65% of hospitals, and primarily treat medical cases. By comparison, private hospitals are in larger communities and account for 35% of hospitals and primarily focus on treating elective cases and conducting procedures. Private hospitals are funded by federal patient subsidies, private insurance, and patient co-payments. Emergency care in Australasia (Australia and New Zealand) mainly occurs in publicly funded, locally run public hospital emergency departments (EDs) (>95%). Most funding (and decision making) is jurisdictional in Australia but with federal grants making 25–40% of the funding, often with key performance indicators (KPIs) and funding agreements, but minimal involvement in program management. In New Zealand, the needs and overall system are similar, but without State governments and with local governance by district health boards.

Australasia has a mature specialty of emergency medicine overseen by the Australasian College for Emergency Medicine (ACEM), with over 1000 Fellows (FACEMs) and 1400 trainees. Many Fellows now work as senior medical administrators, running services and advising governments and others highly involved in medical politics. Most of the population are served by large FACEM-led EDs, with varying mixes of career nonspecialists and trainees. Tertiary EDs have up to 20 full-time employees (FTE) of consultants and 25–35 trainees. Most specialist staffed EDs have at least four FACEM FTEs. Most cities have at least one private ED facility integrated to some degree into service provision, training, and ACEM accreditation. Smaller regional centers often have general practitioner or nurse led services, with varying support from larger centers.

Transportation is a major issue and some patients fly 3500 km to access care within a State. Pre-hospital services are mainly State funded (partial or total) and run by professional ambulance services in urban areas and often volunteer services in regional areas. Regional services are supplemented by aero-retrieval systems such as the iconic, independent, and charitable Royal Flying Doctor Service (RFDS) available to all Australian jurisdictions. Within 250–350 km of major populations, helicopter services provide most retrievals with varying paramedic, nurse, and doctor combinations.

## Access block and crowding

As in most developed countries, decreased acute beds and overcrowded hospitals and EDs have become prevalent in Australia in the past decade. Rates of access block (>8 hours in ED for admitted patients) climbed rapidly in all jurisdictions until 2008–2009.[1] Regular media and published evidence documented poor outcomes, hospital diversions, excessive waits, and ambulance delays.[2,3] In 2009–2010, Western Australia introduced a 4-hour rule whereby patients were expected to be treated and discharged or admitted within 4 hours of arrival (modified from the UK) to drive systematic hospital change. This started in tertiary hospitals in 2010 and all acute hospitals in 2011. Access block was reduced rapidly in tertiary centers, from 50% to 5–15%, with associated improvements in waiting times while indicators of patient safety and rushed care remained stable. However, concerns were raised regarding reduced teaching and training opportunities, increasing staff stresses, and morbidity issues. A new national emergency access target (NEAT) was agreed upon between all Australian jurisdictions in 2011 for stepwise increments to a 90% 4-hour target by 2015. It is too early to predict if this has been successful in driving changes or patient outcomes.

New Zealand (also with FACEM-led EDs) introduced their own 95% by 6-hour targets in 2009 which has been very successful. There are major funded research projects in both countries (more advanced in New Zealand) examining possible benefits and potential downsides of these programs. Hospital and ED crowding resulted in inability of ambulances to offload patients, a very prominent issue in Australia, with administrators, politicians, and the media taking a keen interest. Solutions will probably be similar to those for ED overcrowding.

### Hospital and system capacity

Hospital bed numbers, particularly acute public beds (2.4–2.6 per 1000), are significantly below the recommended averages of the Organisation for Economic Co-operation and Development (OECD) and there has been no significant growth in bed capacity for 15 years. Particularly under-resourced are beds for psychiatric patients, marginalized populations, and older patients with comorbidities. Emergency service demands have increased by around 4% annually, although some States have growth rates of up to 8–10%, and similar or higher admission increases. This reflects an aging population, reduced availability of other services, and rising expectations of care. EDs have responded using short stay units, streaming and frontloading initiatives, plus stronger community-based treatment linkages with demonstrable success.

### Canada

Canada has a universal, publicly funded health care system. The legislative framework is based on the Canadian constitution and federal legislation, but the organization, care delivery, and most financing is in the jurisdiction of the 13 provinces and territories, resulting in 13 similar but distinct health systems. Until 1957, Canada's health care system was very similar to its US counterpart. In that year, the Hospital Insurance and Diagnostic Services Act was established, offering matching federal money to pay 50% of hospital expenditures and thus motivating provinces to put in place national health care insurance. Nine years later, the federal government expanded its funding to share the cost of all physician services.[4] In 1984, the Canada Health Act replaced the two previous laws and articulated the five principles that frame today's provincial insurance systems: portability, accessibility, universality, comprehensiveness, and public administration.[5] Canada's publicly funded systems pay for hospital and ED care, and physician services generally, without co-payments, but are not required to cover out-of-hospital prescription medications or health services delivered by non-physicians. In reality, all provinces have some form of pharmaceutical insurance coverage for the elderly and or those facing catastrophic expenses. Overall, approximately 30% of total health expenditure is paid out-of-pocket or through private insurance.

Today, Canadian physicians remain largely self-employed and fee-for-service has been the dominant payment model, though this is slowly changing. Primary care clinics are almost exclusively privately owned and operated by physicians, but funded on a fee-for-service or blended funding system. This limits the government's influence on provider behavior. Emergency physicians are almost never employees of the hospital and tend to be paid individually or as part of a group contract with the provincial ministry of health based on a blended payment model.

## Emergency department utilization

In 2011, Canadians made 15.8 million visits to the ED, or about 46 visits per 100 population. This is comparable to the United States,[6,7] but an 11-country survey (Australia, France, Germany, the Netherlands, New Zealand, Norway, Sweden, Switzerland, the UK, and the United States) in 2010 found that Canadians had the highest rate of ED utilization, with 44% of those surveyed reporting having used the ED in the prior 2 years.[8] Canadians also reported the lowest rate of accessing primary care services the same day or by a next-day appointment when faced with a minor health problem, and 39% of patients believed that their regular doctor could have addressed the condition for which they last sought emergency care. Though there is good evidence that these low-complexity patients do not cause crowding, the situation translates into long waits for many patients with minor conditions.[9]

## Emergency physician training

Until the mid-1970s, the great majority of physicians working in EDs had trained as general practitioners and no specific training in emergency medicine (EM) was available. The first EM training program in Canada began in 1972 and was followed a decade later by the first specialty board examinations. Around the same period, the College of Family Physicians of Canada also recognized the need for supplemental training in EM and created a 1-year supplemental training program in EM.[10,11] This created two different training streams in Canada: a 5-year EM residency leading to specialty certification (FRCP-EM), and a 2-year residency in family medicine followed by a supplemental year of EM training leading to the CCFP-EM certification. In 2010, there were 593 FRCP-EM trained emergency physicians and 1840 diplomates of the CCFP-EM program in practice in Canada. A total of 2765 family physicians with and without EM certification worked primarily in EDs, and just over 7000 worked there part-time. In recent years, provincial governments have nearly doubled – to nearly 90 – the number of training spots in specialty EM (FRCP-EM), but smaller and more rural EDs, will continue to rely significantly on the work of family physicians for the foreseeable future.[12]

Since its first specialty certification exam in the early 1980s, the scope of practice of EM has evolved. Emergency airway management has become a core competency in EM, along with procedural sedations. Point-of-care ultrasound is also quickly evolving as another core skill of the emergency physician. On the administrative side, ED physicians have taken on administrative roles in pre-hospital care and have taken on leadership roles in the fields of trauma and toxicology.

## Issues in emergency medicine in Canada

Across all provinces, EDs have faced major challenges of overcrowding and geographic accessibility over the last two decades. In a 2010 survey, 31% of Canadians reported waiting more than 4 hours before being treated in the ED, the highest of 11 countries surveyed.[13] In the last few years, many Canadian jurisdictions have launched programs to address crowding. In 2007–2008, the government of Ontario, Canada's largest province, launched an "ER Wait Times Strategy." The program was based on a four-pronged strategy to expand alternatives to emergency visits, increase ED capacity and efficiency, decrease the wait for long-term care beds, and public measuring and reporting of emergency wait times. As of April 2013, the maximal length of stay for 90% of patients had decreased 14%, including over 26% for the most complex patients and 17% for those seeking care for minor conditions.[14] Several other jurisdictions have set targets for wait times in EDs, but there is no agreement nationally on what these targets should be, limiting comparison and collaboration (Table 3.1).[15–17]

While coping with crowding has been a great challenge in larger urban centers, Canada's geography and climate also pose the challenge of providing year-round access to quality emergency care to citizens living in smaller remote communities. In the coastal province of Nova

**Table 3.1** Variation in emergency department length of stay time targets (as of November 2011)

| | Admitions | High Acuity Discharges | Low acuity discharges |
|---|---|---|---|
| | Benchmark/Target | Benchmark/Target | Benchmark/Target |
| Nova Scotia | 8 hours 90th percentile | 8 hours 90th percentile | 4 hours 90th percentile |
| Quebec | 12 hours (mean) | 8 hours (mean)* | |
| Ontario | 8 hours 90th percentile | 8 hours 90th percentile | 4 hours 90th percentile |
| Alberta | 8 hours 90th percentile | 4 hours 90th percentile | |
| British Columbia | 10 hours 75th percentile | 4 hours 75th percentile | 2 hours 75th percentile |

*Applies only to stretcher patients.
*Source*: Courtesy of the Health Quality Council of Alberta [58].

Scotia, small EDs cumulated the equivalent of 795 days of unplanned ED closures, threatening access to emergency care. At the same time, these small departments only averaged one visit per night shift, at an additional cost in physician services of $300 000–700 000 per site annually, a considerable cost the health system. In response to this, alternative models of emergency care are being put in place, including ED staffing with paramedics to supplement the work of nurses and physicians, and a greater integration of air and land medical transport service.[18]

## Denmark

Emergency care services in Denmark are provided through a system of hospital-based EDs, the primary care sector, and the publically run pre-hospital ambulance system. The country is organized into five administrative regions, the governments of which own and operate all public hospitals, fund the primary care system, pre-hospital care, and outpatient specialty care. Most public hospitals have non-overlapping discrete geographic catchment areas for general acute care patients, while some specialty care services are only offered at certain institutions.

Emergency care can be accessed either by:

**1** Contacting one's general practitioner (GP) (during regular office hours) or the GP-run urgent care system (during off hours); or

**2** By calling the universal emergency telephone access number (112) and requesting an ambulance (all hours).

In most parts of the country, patients are discouraged from seeking care directly at a hospital ED without first either contacting the primary care or 112 pre-hospital care systems.

Primary care is universally available to all residents and is delivered by GPs working in private practice, either as solo practitioners or in group practices. Within their local municipality, residents can select a GP, who provides all primary care and also serves as gatekeeper for hospital and specialty care. The GP organization operates a national off-hours urgent care system that includes a telephone call center staffed by GPs, a network of urgent care clinics located in many cases at hospitals, and mobile GPs who make house calls. GPs managing patients with acute complaints can elect to manage the patient's problem over the phone, refer the patient to their own primary care provider, refer the patient to an after-hours urgent care clinic, refer the patient to an ED, arrange for a mobile GP to visit the patient at home, or send an ambulance to take the patient to the hospital.

There is a two-tiered pre-hospital care system – basic life support (BLS) and advanced life support (ALS) – throughout the country. BLS ambulances are staffed mainly by basic level emergency medical technicians (EMTs) who stabilize and transport patients to the nearest ED. Much of the ALS ambulance service consists of mobile units staffed by nurse anesthetists or physicians (usually anesthesiologists, although GPs perform this role in some areas), who, in addition to stabilizing and transporting patients to hospital, also have the option to treat and release patients in the field.

The majority of health care services and virtually all emergency care is publically financed by the national governmental through tax revenues. Approximately 8% of national income tax is earmarked for health care expenditures. Total health care expenditures in 2007 were 9.8% of gross domestic product or $5550 per person annually. GPs are paid under a hybrid capitation (30%) and fee-for-service (70%) agreement between the regional governments and the GP national organization. Hospital-based physicians are employed by the regional government and are paid a fixed salary. Outpatient specialists are paid on a fee-for-service basis.

Historically, hospital-based emergency care throughout Denmark had been delivered via multiple specialty-based EDs located in different parts of the hospital. For example, there would be one ED run by the orthopedic surgery department that would care for trauma patients and minor injuries and another ED run by the internal medicine department that would care for patients with mainly medical problems. These EDs were commonly staffed by junior physicians-in-training with limited supervision by senior physicians from the respective specialties.

In 2007, the National Board of Health released recommendations that the initial management of most acute patients presenting to the hospital be consolidated to a single general purpose ED (*akutafdelinger*), and that this care should be supervised by senior physician specialists. At the same time, a process of consolidating the number of hospitals with EDs was set in motion with the goal of reducing the total number from approximately 40 to 25, based on a planning target of having approximately one general purpose hospital ED per 200 000 inhabitants.[19] While junior physicians-in-training currently still constitute the majority of the ED physician workforce, there is now a small but growing number of senior physicians who have begun working in and providing supervision of ED patient care.

Danes access hospital-based emergency services at an annual rate of 173 visits per 1000 inhabitants and the GP-run urgent care system at an annual rate of 516 contacts per 1000 inhabitants. Most ED visits are compensated at a flat rate if patients are discharged directly to home, regardless of the complexity of the diagnostic evaluation or treatment. If the ED has an associated observation unit within the ED, then there is diagnosis-related group (DRG) -based compensation for those patients that are placed in observation. Only some EDs have observation units. Many ED directors state that the current reimbursement structure does not cover their operating costs, but the hospitals are currently absorbing these costs.[20]

Prior to the recent ED consolidation, primary care or outpatient specialty physicians admitted the majority of acute hospital inpatients directly to a specific inpatient department bypassing the ED. Only about 20% of all acute inpatient admissions came from the ED during the period 2003–2007. Under this model, acute patients referred into the hospital would be seen initially by interns in a receiving area, who would admit the patient to the department requested by the referring physician where the subsequent diagnostic workup and treatment would take place. Little diagnostic evaluation or treatment would take place in the ED, which was reflected in relatively short lengths of stay (LOS) in the ED of less than 2–3 hours and a relatively high rate of inpatient admissions of less than 24–48 hours' duration. Between 10% and 20% of inpatient admissions have LOS of 24 hours or less; 55–65% of inpatient admissions have LOS of 72 hours or less.[21] During the past 10 years, the rate of inpatient discharges has been approximately 17 000 per 100 000 population, which is about 40% higher than the US rate of 12 000 per 100 000 population. The average LOS for inpatient acute care hospital admission in Denmark is 3.5 days compared to 5.6 days in the United States.[22] There is a widespread consensus that many of these short inpatient admissions may be unnecessary, as a high percentage are discharged relatively soon after their first contact with a senior physician on the inpatient service.

Because the 2007 recommendations for ED consolidation are still in the process of being implemented throughout much of the country, the scope of work associated with initial patient management in the ED has yet not changed dramatically and therefore patients' LOS in the ED remains short. As a result, ED crowding has not yet become a significant issue in Denmark. Conversely, there is much discussion about crowding on hospital inpatient wards. Approximately 80% of intensive care units (ICUs) are at 100% occupancy on a regular basis, resulting in frequent transfers between ICUs and cancellations of scheduled surgeries.[23] Similarly, according to the National Board of Health, 30% of the 169 internal medicine departments ran over capacity in 2005, with a total of 78 000 bed days over capacity during that year.[24]

## France

According to the OECD, France ranks high on most measures of health status and is well above the OECD average on a range of key indicators. French citizens have universal health insurance coverage and are free to navigate and be reimbursed for care in a system that includes solo-based fee-for-service private practice for ambulatory care and public hospitals for acute institutional care. The health insurance system grants people access to the registered healthcare professional of their choice. There are no gatekeepers regulating access to specialists and hospitals. The hospitals are paid based on the national tariffs for a stay in hospital. Health care networks have a central role in the French health care system. EM in France has a highly developed pre-hospital Emergency Medical Services (EMS). The particularity of emergency care in France is the multi-tiered pre-hospital EMS and the concept of "stabilize and go."

## Emergency departments

There are two levels of the ED:
- **Level 1**, Service d'Accueil et d'Urgences (SAU), has continuous coverage by surgeons, intensivists, and specialists.
- **Level 2** EDs have certain specialties available only on an "on-call" basis. There are 670 EDs in France with a mean number of 26 000 visits per year. One-third of EDs treat less than 15 000 patients per year and 20% of EDs treat more than 40 000 patients per year.

## Medical schools and emergency medicine

Medical schools are part of free public universities. Emergency physicians and residents from different specialties staff EDs in universities and major teaching hospitals. The length of medical training varies from 8 to 11 years according to specialty and EM is now recognized as a stand-alone specialty.

## Emergency medical service: "stabilize and go"

The EMS (SAMU) was developed in 1968 to coordinate pre-hospital EMS (SMUR for Hospital Mobile and Intensive Care Unit) in the entire country and French overseas departments. In an emergency, French citizens choose between four call numbers closely linked and inter-connected: 17 for police, 18 for fire brigade, 15 for the SAMU call center (managed by hospitals), and 112, the European emergency call number. Calls are received by either SAMU or the fire brigade and then dispatched to the suitable service. These centers cover popula-tions of 200 000–2 000 000, according to administrative regions. There are 101 (http://www.sante.gouv.fr/IMG/pdf/mission_dgos-rapport_modernisation_des_samu-07-2010.pdf) SAMU call centers handling 10 million cases per year (one call per six inhabitants). Thirty percent of calls to the SAMU are managed with information or medical advice, 30% result in the dispatch of a GP on duty, another 30% require sending an ambulance, and 10% involve sending Hospital Mobile Intensive Care Units (HMICU) or sanitary helicopters.[25,26]

## A french concept: "stabilize and go"

SAMU commits the presence of a doctor from the time of the call to the intervention of the HMICU in the field. SAMU's missions are specified by law and ensure that 24 hours a day all calls are answered by trained medical personnel who activate the most appropriate level of response to the emergency call, notify the receiving hospital, participate in the elaboration of mass casualties plans (e.g. bombing, earthquake), and teach emergency medicine.[27]

HMICUs provide medical life support services for the seriously ill and injured on the roads (e.g. resuscitation of patients with multiple trauma) and from France and abroad. SAMU call centers costs 2€ per year per inhabitant and HMICUs costs 10€ per year per inhabitant.

## ED crowding in France and lessons from the heat wave of August 2003

Over the past 10 years, the number of ED visits has increased from 12.2 million visits in 2000 to 17.5 million visits in 2010. EDs became a useful way to access medical care. Emergency calls for the SAMU also increased every year. ED crowding is related to overburdened inpatient facilities, inadequate ED space, insufficient staffing, and inaccessibility of primary care services.[28,29] By French law the ED cannot deny care to patients on the basis of chief complaints and vital signs. Patients requiring vital interventions represent less than 3% of patients using EDs. Moreover, ED patients often report that GPs are not available at night and weekends. In this context, the French government implemented several measures to improve the coordination of healthcare services and EDs and to control the flow of ED visits and to develop primary care units.

In the summer of 2003 a major heat wave occurred in Europe, causing approximately 30 000 deaths, with nearly 15 000 in France.[30] The heat wave was a huge public health disaster in France, when compared with mortality of elderly patients observed during the same periods of the previous 3 years. As a result, French opinion leaders reported that hospitals needed to adopt a multidisciplinary system-wide approach focused on solutions to inpatient capacity constraints. The Société Française de Médecine d'Urgence (SFMU) published recommendations to improve ED crowding which included the regulation of hospitalizations including EDs, observation units, and emergency short stay units, and the interface with general medicine, geriatric, and specialized units (Table 3.2).[31,32]

Table 3.2 Number of emergency departments, HMICU (SMUR) and dispatch centres (SAMU) in France in 2010 (source DRESS: Direction des Recherches etudes evaluations statistiques).

| Hospitals | Public | Private |
|---|---|---|
| Emergency departments | 500 | 170 |
| HMICU (SMUR) | 417 | 9 |
| Dispatch center (SAMU) | 101 | 0 |

## India

In a world population of 7 billion people, almost 20% live in India, making it the largest democracy and the second most populous country in the world.[33] Known as the subcontinent in Asia, India is an up-and-coming economy and in the last two decades has undergone rapid growth, resulting in increased urbanization, motorization, and migration within social classes.[33,34] With this has come many transitions, including those related to the burden of disease. Although infectious diseases still remain a high burden of disease, the incidence and prevalence of noncommunicable diseases and injuries are on the rise and this trend is expected to continue over the next 25 years.[35] In fact, the leading causes of mortality in India are cardiovascular disease and injuries, in both urban and rural areas.[36] To deal with this changing burden of disease, the health care system needs to adapt and improve its scope of care. For this reason, EM is one of the fastest growing specialties in the Indian health sector.

In India, care is provided in two arenas: the public and the private sectors. In the public sector, the services are free, but there are often long waiting times and the quality of the care provided is variable. In the public EDs, there are usually medical officers in training in all different specialties working in the ED and there is no formal triage system. In the private sector, the quality of care seems to be better, but again there is a lack of formal triage systems, and patients are required to pay out of pocket before services are rendered. In both sectors, there are no dedicated trauma surgeons, with orthopedists generally leading any major traumas. There are only a handful of major trauma centers in the country and the pre-hospital care system is weak. The existing EMS systems are largely private, often with personnel that are not trained in pre-hospital care, and who do not provide medical care en route. Because they are private and patients have to pay upfront, people often come to the ED by either private car or public transportation, such as auto-rickshaws, flatbed trucks, or taxis.[37,38]

Currently, there are many types of educational programs specific to EM in India. First, there are those offered as postgraduate Masters programs offered by different private universities, often in private hospitals. There are also short certificate courses that provide some EM training to those who are already working in EDs. For these programs, there are no standards in length of training or curriculum, the Medical College of India (MCI) does not officially recognize them, and therefore graduates from these programs are unable to work as EM faculty at government hospitals.[37]

In 2009, the MCI recognized EM as a specialty. As of May 2012, there were a total of 25 seats available at different government-run hospitals officially recognized to provide postgraduate training in EM.[39] Of these, 16 positions were opened up in 2012. Furthermore, to promote EM in India, there are currently five national EM societies, who host national EM conferences in addition to carrying out advocacy work.[39]

Overall, India is on the right track to improving its emergency medical care services. However, there is still room for improvement and growth. First and foremost, the MCI needs to open more EM training positions because the current number is not nearly enough to expand the field at a rate appropriate for the country's needs. In addition, EM also needs to be incorporated into the medical school curriculum. For pre-hospital care, there need to be appropriate training programs in place and better alignment of services so that those patients who truly need pre-hospital services can access them without delay or significant cost. On the preparedness side, the disaster systems should be improved so that they can be carried out more effectively and efficiently. Finally, there needs to be greater emphasis on injury care, given its high prevalence in the country, not only from the treatment perspective, but also for prevention.

India has shown itself to be a progressive country and a leader in its part of the world. As evidenced by the rapidly growing field of EM in the country, it has shown that it recognizes its importance. With continued emphasis on improving emergency care and advocacy by current emergency medical providers in India, there is hope for the future.

## Iran

The development of EM as a medical specialty has been a long journey but has resulted in the acknowledgement of the essential role of EM in the health care system in Iran. Today, well-established and functional EMS is seen as one of the critical components of Iran's healthcare system. Three decades ago, Iran joined the ranks of those countries with a functional EMS network.

The Islamic Republic of Iran has a population of 75 million, living in a $636\ 372\ mi^2$ area located in the geographic region commonly identified as the Middle East. Iran's healthcare system is composed of regional primary care clinics and public hospitals providing primary to tertiary care throughout the country. In addition, many corporate and privately owned facilities provide healthcare services, mainly in the large cities. Emergency and urgent care services are provided through EDs at larger hospitals. EDs are mainly staffed by emergency physicians or specialists from other disciplines dedicated exclusively to EM practice. There are a growing number of EM residency programs that provide training for physicians with a commitment to staff the public hospital EDs. Increasing the number of EDs, training emergency physicians and nurses, and facilitating emergency services gained the highest priority in the national health care system during the past 10 years. Likewise, the emergency care system sponsored by the state has received more resources to provide emergency services for the majority of Iran's citizens.

The basis for Iran's implementation of emergency care comes from Articles 3, 29, and 43 of Iran's constitution, which state that the government of Iran must meet the basic needs of the public, which includes education and healthcare. Overall, the guiding principle behind Iran's emergency care system is centralization. Universities and government hospitals provide the means and materials by which Iranian citizens receive emergency care. The government also provides a common emergency communication number, "Emergency 115," in accordance with the basic principles of EMS worldwide. Emergency 115 is only used for contacting the EMS, as it will only communicate with EM centers. Emergency 115 services are coordinated by Communication and Operations Directing Centers (CODC), which also act as the coordinator of emergency bases and stations. All units that are activated by the emergency 115 system must take appropriate measures as determined by CODC after a call for assistance is received. The communication centers are individually located in provincial centers that have a population of more than 250 000.[40]

In 1999, Iranian authorities accepted the Anglo-American model for emergency care delivery and training. In 2001, Iran began academic training of emergency physicians. The role of emergency care in Iran was defined as "improvement and development of the services to treat victims of accidents and sudden diseases, as well as, to address other medical emergencies."[41] In order to accomplish the goal of timely treatment of patients, the emergency care system is composed of several components, primarily emergency ambulances and EDs.

Promotion of the emergency care system in Iran consists of investments to improve patient transportation, expand the number of facilities, and focus on educational activities for emergency care providers. With the cooperation of the World Bank, the Ministry of Health and Medical Education was able to obtain a total of 500 locally constructed ambulances. With the goal of improving accessibility to emergency care across Iran, further improvements in pre-hospital services include expectations for high quality services, encouraging technologic upgrades to enhance communication, and the creation of treatment plans and guidelines for emergency care.[42,43] Such efforts have significantly improved the quality of care and delivery of services for trauma patients, but there are still challenges to overcome. Iran's emergency care system still struggles with obstacles such as manpower, education, insufficient transport vehicles, communication, and traffic.

In 2001, the first group of EM residents was selected among a group of interested physicians by way of a national residency examination. The impetus for the start of an EM training program came from a visit to the United States by a core group of Iranian specialists observing the current practice of emergency care. Since that first class, the Tehran University of Medical Sciences became the second university after Iran Medical University to start its own EM residency program in 2004. The Iranian Society of Emergency Medicine holds an international EM conference in Tehran on an annual basis which usually attracts over 1000 participants.[41,44]

As the emergency care system in Iran has evolved, Iran has had to confront many of the traditional problems faced by countries with a transitional level of EM development. Foremost among these are financial constraints, as significant funds are needed to construct more advanced clinical facilities, run faculty and academic training programs, and participate in medical research. There are also insufficient numbers of inpatient bed in public hospitals and a limited availability of ancillary services which adversely affects the current ED services in many hospitals.[45] Further complications hindering efforts to improve the emergency care system is the friction between various medical specialties and where the newly fashioned EM specialty belongs. Despite these hurdles, the increase of EM professionals trained in Iran can be taken as a positive sign for the future of emergency care in Iran.

## Japan

### Pre-hospital care in Japan
A characteristic of pre-hospital care in Japan is that the EM system is completely sponsored by the Ministry of Internal Affairs and Communications. Since legislation establishing the ambulance service in 1963, all citizens can call an ambulance by dialling 119 at no charge. The number of emergency calls increased dramatically from less than 300 000 dispatches in 1963 to 5 463 682 in 2011. This increase is not only because of aging of the society but also the increasing demand by Japanese citizens for quality emergency medical care. As of 2011 there are 4927 ambulance teams and 59 650 EMTs nationwide. A response time from emergency call to arrival at the scene is 8 minutes on average and the time from emergency call to arrival at the hospital averages 37 minutes. Notably, these time periods have been getting longer in the past decade because of the increasing number of dispatches.[46,47]

Until the 1980s, Japanese pre-hospital ambulances were not equipped with advanced skills such as automated external defibrillators (AED), airway devices, and drugs. Emergency life-saving technicians (ELST), comparable with paramedics in the United States, were first created by law in 1991 and have gradually increased in number to 21 268. However, the advanced skills by ELSTs are limited to care for cardiac arrest patients. The government hopes to expand the skills to pre-arrest care such as saline transfusion to shock patients, inhalation of beta stimulants to asthmatic patients, and measurement of blood glucose for hypoglycemic patients.

## Hospital care

In Japan, there are 3914 emergency hospitals and 367 clinics (total 4281) divided into three tiers. The primary tier is a medical facility without hospital beds, the second tier is a medical facility with hospital beds, and the third tier is an emergency medical service center (EMSC), where any patient with a life-threatening condition is accepted 24/7. An EMSC is a division of a critical care unit in a hospital focused on emergency patients. Most hospitals with an EMSC have inpatient beds and also function as second tier facilities. EMSCs are a unique characteristic of the Japanese emergency care system and were founded in 1977 and funded by the government. Transported patients are triaged by ambulance teams and only those with life-threatening vital signs are transported to an EMSC. In 2012, there were 245 EMSCs across Japan. The government requirement for the approval of an EMSC is that the facility must have an ICU dedicated to emergency patients with 20 beds and full-time doctors. Staffing of EMSC varies widely from a few to more than 30 physicians.

A specialty board for EM was founded by Japanese Association for Acute Medicine (JAAM) in 1973. JAAM supplies board certified physicians to emergency hospitals nationwide but it is acknowledged that there is a shortage of EM boarded physicians, with only 3374 in 2012. There are a total of 466 hospitals, including EMSCs, with more than two full-time emergency physicians and approved as training hospitals for emergency physicians. The remaining emergency hospitals are without emergency physicians and emergency patients are managed on a multispecialty model, where nonemergency physicians rotate to care for emergency patients at night. Recently, US style EM where emergency physicians care for both life-threatening and nonacute patients, has been introduced to Japan and more than 150 JAAM-affiliated hospitals have implemented this type of EM as of 2007.[48]

## ED visits

Japanese EDs see about 25 million visits annually; however, the precise records for patients who visited the EDs are limited to those who were transported by ambulances and it is estimated that there are about 4 walk-in patients for every patient transported by ambulance. Statistics of nationwide ambulance service records show that severity of medical conditions of transported victim are distributed as follows: mild 50.4%, who mostly are discharged home; moderate 38.4%; severe 9.6%; and fatal 1.5%. This classification is not based on triage by expert nurses but on documents written by physicians caring for emergency patients when they arrived at ED.[49]

# Singapore

The population of Singapore is 4 657 542, with a life expectancy of 79 years for men and 83 years for women. There are 15 physicians per 10 000 people and infant mortality is 2.3 per 1000 births, one of the lowest in the world. The government health expenditures as a percentage of total government expenditures was 7.2% in 2007. There are seven public hospitals in Singapore: five acute general hospitals, a women's and children's hospital, and a psychiatric hospital. The general hospitals provide multidisciplinary acute inpatient and specialist outpatient services and 24-hour EDs. In addition, there are six national specialty centers for cancer, cardiac, eye, skin, neuroscience, and dental care. In addition, there are seven privately owned hospitals that provide health care services.

## Health care financing

Singapore offers universal health care coverage to their citizens, with a financing system anchored on the twin philosophies of individual responsibility and affordable health care for all (government subsidies through taxation). The government has established the 3M framework of Medisave, Medishield, and Medifund which combines individual responsibility and is overlaid with government funding, particularly to provide a safety net to support the health needs of low income earners and poorer individuals. Compulsory participation in Medisave accounts covers inpatient services, hospitals, physicians' fees, surgical procedures, immunizations, screenings, family planning services, and psychiatric care, with some limits to usage. It is financed through medical savings accounts, and income. Medishield is a high-deductible catastrophic insurance plan for those under 70 years old. All Medisave patients are enrolled but can opt out (88% enroll). Medifund is an endowment fund set up by the Singapore government to assist those in financial hardship in funding their medical needs. Qualification for Medifund provision is means tested, based on an individual's financial circumstances at the time of application.[50,51] In addition to individuals self-financing through Medisave and Medishield, a significant portion of workers (and their dependents) are covered by private health insurance. Private health insurance, which is often funded by employers on behalf of employees, covers a diverse range of medical expenses that are not typically reimbursed under the 3M system.

Under Medisave, patients are able to choose their providers and pay directly for the services at the point of delivery. There are 13 public hospitals, over 2000 private medical clinics, and 15 government polyclinics (similar to community health centers in the United States) which provide health care services.[52] Singapore has a mixed medical care delivery system. In acute care, the public sector providers make up nearly 80% of the market while private providers dominate the primary care sector, also with nearly 80% of the market. Eighty percent of hospital care in Singapore is provided by public hospitals, where the government puts price caps on all services and procedures.[53] Accident and emergency (A&E) services are subsidized by the Singapore government at 50% as a flat attendance fee imposed regardless of nationality.

### Practice of EM in Singapore

From 2001 to 2010, there was a 52% increase in annual A&E attendances (Figure 3.1) while the population of Singapore went from 4 to 5 million, a 25% increase. In 2010, about 850 000 ED visits were treated at seven public sector EDs. This was a 4.6% increase over the previous year and it is envisaged that ED visits will hit the million mark by 2014 (Figure 3.1).

Singapore adopted a four-level patient acuity status triage system with P1 being the most severe cases and P4 the non-urgent cases. About 6% of cases are P1, 35–40% are P2, and slightly over 50% are P3. The preponderance of P3 ambulatory cases divert scarce ED resources from the more seriously ill P1 and P2 patients. Social interventions were able to reduce nonemergency P3 cases by 40% over the 12-year period (Figure 3.2).

### The silver tsunami

According to the Committee on Aging Issues, one in every five residents of Singapore will be a senior by 2030. Senior patients present with higher

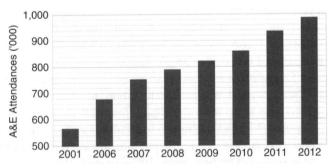

**Figure 3.1** Annual emergency department attendances (public sector hospitals only), singapore. Data for 2006–2012 from http://www.singstat.gov.sg/publications /publications_and_papers/reference/yearbook_2013/excel/topic21.xls: Table 21.2, hospital admissions and public sector outpatient attendances.

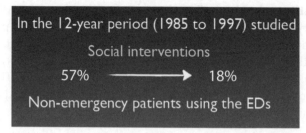

In the 12-year period (1985 to 1997) studied

Social interventions

57% ⟶ 18%

Non-emergency patients using the EDs

**Figure 3.2** Proportion of non-emergency social P3 cases reduced by social interventions. Data from Anantharaman V. Impact of healthcare system interventions on emergency department utilization and overcrowding in singapore. Int J emerg med. 2008;1:11–20.

acuity, are more likely to arrive by ambulance, consume more time and resources, and are more likely to be admitted. They are also more likely to reattend at the ED following discharge. Presenting with multiple chronic diseases and comorbidities, with atypical presentations as the rule rather than the exception, and sometimes scant social support, Singapore needs to reconsider if the traditional fast-paced "see-and-treat-or-admit" role is sufficient to meet the needs of an aging population.

## Towards integrated care

The EM community in Singapore is looking for solutions outside of EDs and hospitals. It sees its new role in care coordination and optimizing the utilization of community resources. This needs to be addressed at a systems level, involving changes in health-seeking behavior of patients, review of current EM practices, financial incentives or disincentives, engaging the community health partners, and patient education and training.

### "From disease to wellness"

It is desirable to keep Singaporeans healthy so that they do not come into the acute health care system. This will be done by increasing the role of the Health Promotion Board's prevention and education efforts, detecting and treating diseases early through health screening in GP clinics and in the community, and restructuring hospitals to help the frail elderly and patients with chronic diseases manage their medical conditions better.

### "From provider to patient"

Seamless care beyond the hospital across a network of primary care and intermediate and long-term care providers requires the various parties to look beyond organizational boundaries, professional cultures, and business models to structure care based on what is trouble-free, patient-centric, and the best system for the patient.

**"From institution to home"**
The priority of Singaporean health care institutions is to heal patients so that they can go home. Health care institutions must help patients maintain contact with their families by explaining the patient's care plans and goals, facilitating family visitations, and home leave arrangements. These institutions also address gaps in service planning, capabilities, and resources that currently hinder patients from returning home.

**"From isolation to integration"**
This starts with restructuring of services so that each provider does not deliver care in an isolated way, but rather with a multidisciplinary approach to patient care management.

To meet these goals the Society and Chapter of Emergency Medicine of Singapore set up a working group in 2011 to look into writing a White Paper – "The State of Emergency Medicine in Singapore."

## United Kingdom

Despite universal coverage, a strong network of GPs, and a variety of sites for unscheduled care, such as walk-in centers and after-hour GP clinics, demands on EDs in England continue to rise. Attendances increased from 14.2 million in 1998–1999 to 21.3 million in 2010–2011.[54] Until recently, EDs (formerly known as accident and emergency departments, A&Es) were infamous for their "corridors of shame": patients lying on stretchers for 12 hours or more waiting for admission to hospital and reception areas filled with patients waiting 6–8 hours to see a physician. In 2000, the new Labour government promised to change this. "By 2004, no-one should be waiting more than four hours in accident and emergency from arrival to admission, transfer or discharge."[55] The 4-hour target was implemented in a graduated fashion. Initially, 90% of patients had to be seen and either discharged or admitted (and out of the ED) within 4 hours, then 94%, 96%, and 98%. Hospitals that met the target at each stage received £100 000 ($150 000). Target performance was reported publicly on the Department of Health website and hospital leadership (not the EDs) were made responsible for meeting the target, with an implication that jobs were on the line. The National Health Service (NHS) established an Emergency Services Collaborative which brought representatives of hospitals together to discuss and encourage process changes to improve flow within the ED and the hospital, but EDs were free to determine how to change their processes to meet the target. Many EDs adopted streaming (separation of major and minor patients), "see and treat," and eliminated formal triage. Most added a clinical decision unit where patients requiring more than 4-hour evaluation, but not admission, could be watched prior to discharge. Investigations were started earlier, more senior ED consultants were hired, and ED physicians were given more admitting rights to other services. However, to solve the wait for admitted patients, the rest of the hospital had to find ways to create beds, including improving its admission planning and discharge processes, which many UK hospitals still struggle with.

Quarterly Department of Health data suggest that one-third to half of hospitals failed to meet the 4-hour target for 98% of patients, but the bulk of hospitals met the target for 95–97% of patients, and nearly all hospitals reported meeting it for at least 90%.[56] Close observers would agree that conditions markedly improved. However, there were concerns that some degree of cheating may have been going on, perhaps with back-timing discharges and admissions by a few (or more) minutes, to register the discharges within 4 hours.[57] The safety of the 4-hour limit has also not been determined. It is unknown if patients who might benefit from additional time in the ED for better planning, testing, and treatment are put at risk by this time limit. Concerns have also been raised about whether patients are treated quickly and appropriately in the ED but rushed out, only to find themselves on an available, but inappropriate, ward or to then undergo a long wait for evaluation by an inpatient team, delaying care that could have been received sooner had they remained in the ED.

Despite lack of definitive evidence of the target's benefit or harm (and more likely a mixture), the Conservative government abolished the target entirely in April 2011, a move that has emergency providers concerned about backsliding to the "bad old days."

## References

1 Richardson DB, Kelly AM, Kerr D. Prevalence of access block in Australia 2004–2008. Emerg Med Australas. 2009;21:472–8.
2 Richardson DB. Increase in patient mortality at 10 days associated with emergency department overcrowding. Med J Aust. 2006;184:213–6.
3 Sprivulis PC, Da Silva JA, Jacobs IG, Frazer AR, Jelinek GA. The association between hospital overcrowding and mortality among patients admitted via Western Australian emergency departments. Med J Aust. 2006;184:208–12.
4 Government of Canada HC. Canada's Health Care System. Health Canada, 2011. Available at: http://www.hc-sc.gc.ca/hcs-sss/pubs/system-regime/2011-hcs-sss/index-eng.php (accessed 26 November 2013).
5 Loi canadienne sur la santé. (1985). L.R.C., 1985, ch. C-6.
6 Canadian Institute for Health Information (CIHI). (2012) Highlights of 2010–2011 Inpatient Hospitalizations and Emergency Department Visits. Ottawa, Ont.: CIHI.
7 Centers for Disease Control and Prevention (CDC). FASTSTATS. Hospital Utilization. Available at: http://www.cdc.gov/nchs/fastats/hospital.htm (accessed 26 November 2013).

8 Leatherman ST, Sutherland K. Canadian Health Services Research Foundation, Canadian Patient Safety Institute, Canadian Institute for Health Information, Statistics Canada. Quality of Healthcare in Canada: A Chartbook. Ottawa, Ont.: Canadian Health Services Research Foundation, 2010.

9 Schull MJ, Kiss A, Szalai JP. The effect of low-complexity patients on emergency department waiting times. Ann Emerg Med. 2007;49(3):257–264.

10 Arnold JL. International emergency medicine and the recent development of emergency medicine worldwide. Ann Emerg Med. 1999;33(1):97–103.

11 Steiner IP. Emergency medicine practice and training in Canada. Canadian Med Assoc J. 2003;168(12):1549–50.

12 Canadian Resident Matching Service (CaRMS). Reports and Statistics, 2012 Match Reports. Available at: http://www.carms.ca/eng/operations_R1reports_12_e.shtml (accessed 26 November 2013).

13 Schoen C, Osborn R. 2010 International Health Policy Survey in Eleven Countries. The Commonwealth Fund, 2010.

14 Government of Ontario Ministry of Health and Long-term Care. Ontario Wait Times Strategy. http://www.health.gov.on.ca/en/public/programs/waittimes/strategy.aspx (accessed 26 November 2013).

15 Coleman J, Sutherland-Boal A, Chase M, McCurdy G. Emergency Department Pay for Performance Pilot.Vancouver, B.C.: Vancouver Coastal Health. Available at: http://acaho.org/docs_new/Patient%20Flow/12-VCH-Emergency%20Department%20Pay%20for%20Performance%20(Final).pdf (accessed 26 November 2013).

16 Alberta Health and Wellness. Becoming the Best: Alberta's 5-Year Health Action Plan 2010–2015. Edmonton, Alb: Government of Alberta, 2011.

17 MSSS. Rapport annuel de gestion 2010–2011 du ministère de la Santé et des Services sociaux. Quebec City, Que.: Quebec Government, 2011.

18 Ross J. The patient journey through emergency care in Nova Scotia: a prescription for new medicine. Halifax, Nova Scotia: Provincial Advisor on Emergency Care, 2010.

19 Styrket Akutberedskab – planlægningsgrundlag for the regionale sundshedsvæsen. Copenhagen: Sundhedsstyrelsen, 2007.

20 Anderson PD, et al. Report on the Emergency Care Delivery System in Region Nordjylland. Boston, MA: Harvard Medical Faculty Physicians, 2008.

21 Kristensen S, Johnsen SP, Madsen BE, Anderson PD. Forekomst og beskrivelse af akutte indlæggelser og skadestuebesøg i Region Nordjylland og Midtjylland: Klinisk Epidemiologisk Afdeling, Aarhus Universitet, 2009.

22 OECD. Health at a Glance 2009: OECD Indicators, OECD Publishing, 2009.

23 Lippert A, Espersen K, Antonsen K, Joensen H, Waldau TE, Larsen KM. Capacity in Danish intensive care units. A national survey of capacity, cancellations and transfers of critically ill patients [in Danish]. Ugeskr Læger. 2007;169:712–6.

24 Schmidt AL. Dødssyge ender på hospitalsgangen. Politiken, 2007.

25 French Society of Emergency Medicine (SFMU). Situation of Emergency Departments in France. Available at: http://www.sfmu.org/documents/ressources/referentiels/Aval_SU_SFMU_mai_2005.pdf (accessed 26 November 2013).

26 Szmajer M, Rodriguez P, Sauval P, Charetteur MP, Derossi A, Carli P. Medical assistance during commercial airline flights: analysis of 11 years experience of the

Paris Emergency Medical Service (SAMU) between 1989 and 1999. Resuscitation. 2001;50(2):147–51.

27  Masmejean EH, Faye A, Alnot JY, Mignon AF. Trauma care systems in France. Injury. 2003;34(9):669–73.

28  Somme D, Lazarovici C, Dramé M, Blanc P, Lang PO, Gauvain JB, et al. The geriatric patient: use of acute geriatrics units in the emergency care of elderly patients in France. Arch Gerontol Geriatr. 2011;52(1):40–5.

29  Baubeau B, Deville A, Joubert M. Emergency department visits in France from 1990 to 1998, a growing need for non-urgent visits [in French]. DREES, Etudes et Résultats. 2000;72:1–8.

30  Belmin J, Auffray JC, Berbezier C, Boirin P, Mercier S, de Reviers B, et al. Level of dependency: a simple marker associated with mortality during the 2003 heatwave among French dependent elderly people living in the community or in institutions. Age Ageing. 2007;36(3):298–303.

31  Claessens YE, Taupin P, Kierzek G, Pourriat JL, Baud M, Ginsburg C, et al. How emergency departments might alert for prehospital heat-related excess mortality? Critical Care. 2006;10(6):R156.

32  Gentile S, Vignally P, Durand AC, Gainotti S, Sambuc R, Gerbeaux P. Non urgent patients in the emergency department? A French formula to prevent misuse. BMC Health Serv Res. 2010;10:66.

33  Government of India, Ministry of Health and Family Welfare (MOH) 2011. Annual Report to the People on Health. Ministry of Health and Family Welfare, New Delhi, India. Available at: http://mohfw.nic.in/WriteReadData/l892s/6960144509Annual%20Report%20to%20the%20People%20on%20Health.pdf (accessed 26 November 2013).

34  Government of India, Ministry of Health and Family Welfare (MOH) 2005. Background papers: Burden of Disease in India. National Commission on Macroeconomics and Health, Ministry of Health and Family Welfare. New Delhi, India. Available at: http://www.who.int/macrohealth/action/Report%20of%20the%20National%20Commission.pdf (accessed 26 November 2013).

35  Jacob JT, Dandona L, Sharma VP, Kakkar M. India: towards universal health coverage 1. Continuing challenge of infectious diseases in India. Lancet. 2011;377:252–69.

36  Patel V, Chatterji S, Chisholm D, Ebrahim S, Gopalakrishna G, Mathers C, et al. India: towards universal health coverage 3. Chronic diseases and injuries in India. Lancet. 2011;377:413–28.

37  Das AK, Gupta SB, Joshi SR, Aggarwal P, Murmu LR, Bhoi S, et al. White paper on academic emergency medicine in India: INDO-US joint working group (JWG). J Assoc Physicians India. 2008;56:789–98.

38  Alagappan K, Cherukuri K, Narang V, Kwiatkowski T, Rajagopalan A. Early development of emergency medicine in Chennai (Madras). India Ann Emerg Med. 1998;32(5):604–8.

39  EmergencyMedicine. Available at; http://www.emergencymedicine.in/current/articles.php?article_id=56 (accessed 26 November 2013).

40  Bahrami MA, Maleki A, Ranjbar Ezzatabadi M, Askari R, Ahmadi Tehrani GH. Pre-hospital emergency medical services in developing countries: a case study about EMS response time in Yazd, Iran. Iran Red Crescent Med J. 2011;13(10):735–8.

41 Smith JP, Shokoohi H, Holliman JC. The search for common ground: developing emergency medicine in Iran. Acad Emerg Med. 2007;14:457–62.

42 Djalali A, Castren M, Hosseinijenab V, Khatib M, Ohlen G, Kurland L. Hospital Incident Command System (HICS) performance in Iran; decision making during disasters. Scand J Trauma Resusc Emerg Med. 2012;20:14.

43 Hassani SA, Moharari RS, Sarvar M, Nejati A, Khashayar P. Helicopter emergency medical service in Tehran, Iran: a descriptive study. Air Med J. 2012;31(6):294–7.

44 Pines JM, Hilton JA, Weber EJ, Alkemade AJ, et.al. International perspectives on emergency department crowding. Acad Emerg Med. 2011;18(12):1358–70.

45 Hatamabady HR. Causes of length of stay in a typical crowded emergency department of a teaching hospital in Tehran capital city. Ann Emerg Med. 2008;52:S131.

46 Ministry of Internal Affairs and Communication. Current status of emergency and rescue 2011 [In Japanese]. Available at: http://www.fdma.go.jp/neuter/topics /houdou/h23/2312/231216_1houdou/02_mokuji.pdf (accessed 16 December 2013).

47 Hori S. EMS in Japan. In: Tintinalli JE, Cameron P, Holliman CJ (eds.) EMS: A Practical Global Guide Book. PMPH-USA, Shelton, 2010: pp.54–66.

48 Yamashita M, Akashi K, Ohta B, et al. Implementation of US style emergency medicine in JAAM affiliated hospitals. J Jpn Ass Acute Med. 2008;19:416–23.

49 Hori S. Emergency medicine in Japan. Keio J Med. 2010;59:131–9.

50 Pauly M. Medical savings accounts in Singapore: what can we know? J Health Polit Policy Law. 2001;26:727–32.

51 Barr MD. Medical savings accounts in Singapore: a critical inquiry. J Health Polit Policy Law. 2001;26:709–26.

52 Massaro TA, Wong Y-N. Medical Savings Accounts: The Singapore experience. Dallas, TX: National Centre for Policy Analysis, Policy Report No. 203, April 1996. Available at: http://www.ncpa.org/pub/st203 (accessed 13 December 2013).

53 Meng-Kim L. Health care systems in transition II. Singapore, Part I. An overview of health care systems in Singapore. J Public Health Med. 1998;20(1):16–22.

54 Department of Health (UK). http://webarchive.nationalarchives.gov.uk /20110203014133/http://www.dh.gov.uk/en/Publicationsandstatistics/Statistics /Performancedataandstatistics/AccidentandEmergency/DH_087973(accessed 13 December 2013).

55 The NHS Plan: a plan for investment, plan for reform. July, 2000. http://pns.dgs.pt /files/2010/03/pnsuk1.pdf (accessed 12 December 2013).

56 Department of Health (UK) Performance Data and Statistics. http:// webarchive.nationalarchives.gov.uk/20110203014133/http://www.dh.gov.uk/en /Publicationsandstatistics/Statistics/Performancedataandstatistics/Accidentand Emergency/DH_079085 (accessed 12 December 2010).

57 Locker T, Mason S. Analysis of the distribution of time that patients spend in Emergency Departments. BMJ. 2005;330:1188–9.

58 Affleck A, Parks P, Drummond A, Rowe BH, Ovens HJ. Emergency department overcrowding and access block. CJEM. 2013;15:359–70.

# PART 2

# Technology in emergency care

# CHAPTER 4

# Human factors in emergency care

**Raj M. Ratwani[1], A. Zach Hettinger[2], and
Rollin J. Fairbanks[1,3,4]**

[1]*MedStar Institute for Innovation, National Center for Human Factors in
Healthcare, USA*
[2]*Department of Emergency Medicine, Georgetown University
School of Medicine, National Center for Human Factors in
Healthcare, USA*
[3]*National Center for Human Factors in Healthcare, MedStar Institute for
Innovation, Department of Emergency Medicine, USA*
[4]*Industrial Systems Engineering, University at Buffalo, USA*

The field of human factors engineering (HFE), also known as ergonomics, is concerned with understanding the capabilities and characteristics of humans and applying this knowledge to improve the tools, machines, and systems with which humans interact.[1] HFE seeks to improve human performance and safety by focusing on the cognitive and physical capabilities of the "user" as they operate in their work environment, and using this information to inform system design. Knowledge of cognitive capabilities includes understanding attention processes, memory demands, perception, information processing, and decision-making. Physical capabilities include understanding the anatomy, physiology, and biomechanics of the user. Given the focus on both cognitive and physical capabilities, HFE is a multidisciplinary field that draws from psychology, engineering, and anthropometry.

This chapter reviews common methods used in HFE and the application of HFE to health care with a focus on emergency medicine. Specific topics covered include workflow, overcrowding, teamwork, health information technology, task interruptions, and clinical decision-making. While HFE has an extensive history in domains such as aviation and nuclear energy, the application of HFE in health care is still in its early stages.

*Emergency Care and The Public's Health*, First Edition.
Edited by Jesse M. Pines, Jameel Abualenain, James Scott and Robert Shesser.
© 2014 John Wiley & Sons, Ltd. Published 2014 by John Wiley & Sons, Ltd.

## Human factors engineering methods

The application of HFE theories and principles to a particular domain requires an understanding of the user's goals and how the user interacts with their surroundings to accomplish these goals. In order to develop a more complete representation of how work is performed, a systems approach is used when examining the emergency medicine providers' interactions with the environment, people, and devices within the environment.[2] A variety of qualitative and quantitative methods are used to gain an understanding of these interactions within the environment. Three common human factors methods are observational analysis, task analysis, and simulation.

### Observational analysis

This method was originally derived from ethnography and involves documenting the interactions of the worker in their actual work environment (*in situ*). Observations may be conducted to gain a general understanding of how health care providers interact with their work environment. This descriptive understanding may then be used to inform the development of new technology or tools. For example, an HFE expert may shadow an emergency physician to gain a detailed understanding of the discharge process from both workflow and cognitive standpoints. The emergency department information system (EDIS) can then be designed to present the important data at the right time, and provide the correct functions in the right order. This type of optimized system can lead to improvements in both safety and efficiency.

For validation or to compare systems, prospective observational studies may be conducted by having trained researchers observe and systematically document particular user behaviors and interactions, after which the data are analyzed. By conducting these observations before and after a specific intervention or by using controls, the effect of the intervention can be quantitatively evaluated.

### Task analysis

This method involves developing a very detailed description of the specific user processes as they interact within a system (such as an emergency department (ED)), or with system components (such as a medical device or health IT system). Understanding tasks at this level of detail allows optimization for efficiency, and minimization of any potential for errors, by matching these processes to human capabilities.[3] There are several types of task analyses that can be conducted including hierarchical and cognitive task analyses.[4] In hierarchical task analysis the focus is on the specific set of steps and processes, and the contingencies among these steps, that a user must perform in order to accomplish a task.

Cognitive task analysis focuses on the mental processes of the user, such as reasoning and problem-solving, as he/she works to accomplish a task.

Task analysis may be performed by observing users in their work environment, conducting semi-structured interviews where users are asked about their tasks and how they accomplish these tasks, or by conducting focus groups. Usability studies, which serve to evaluate the overall functionality of a software tool or system, often rely on task analysis methods.

## Simulation

Although simulation is generally thought of as a training tool, it is also a powerful approach to studying human factors in the ED. Both computer and live simulation offer the opportunity to collect data on specific tasks or procedures that may be rare in an actual environment, introduce system changes, and determine the effectiveness of the changes. For example, simulation can be used to systematically examine how effective workflow manipulations are in reducing the rate of provider interruptions in the ED.

For HFE research to be as effective in health care as it has been in industries such as aviation and nuclear energy, medical simulation must be leveraged to a larger degree. The complexities of the collecting data and performing experimental tests during the actual delivery of health care is very challenging and present serious challenges to human factors researchers and simulation provides a good alternative method to evaluate a new technology design or changes to workflow process.

## Workflow

The ability to treat patients safely while efficiently moving them through the ED necessitates a well-designed system. " Workflow" refers to both the way in which health care workers navigate through the physical space and to the specific work processes and steps that must be accomplished in order to complete a particular task or goal.[5,6] Studying work processes requires an understanding of the mental steps that must be accomplished, the interaction with computer systems and other machines, and intradepartmental communication. While methods such as Lean and Six Sigma focus on improving efficiency by reducing waste, human factors methods focus on supporting the cognitive needs of the worker, and building redundancy where necessary as a critical safety function.[7–10]

The successful use of human factors analysis in other high risk industries can provide examples for emergency medicine's quest to reduce errors and hazards.[11] Many health care adminstrators take for granted the incredible complexity of the clinical environment and how well their workforce navigate the system and prevent harm to patients.[12] All stages in the patient's journey through the ED can benefit from human factors analysis.[13,14]

The introduction of new technologies into the ED requires an analysis of how the technology influences workflow to ensure that the needs of the user are met and that no new errors are introduced. For example, the addition of health information technology (health IT) can have an effect on workflow, including how staff communicates and the way that teams operate; health IT is discussed in greater detail later.[15,16]

## Overcrowding

Researchers have documented the negative effects of overcrowding on patient safety and patient satisfaction.[17] Overcrowding is associated with increased in-hospital mortality, increased rates of medical errors, and increased rates of patients both leaving the hospital without being seen and signing out against medical advice.[18]

Researchers have addressed the overcrowding problem by examining the influence of admission and discharge procedures on overcrowding.[19] They have concluded that a systems approach that looks at the entire hospital, not just the ED, is required to address the ED overcrowding problem.[19,20] A systems approach can be used to identify multiple factors that need to be aligned in order to control overcrowding and multiple solutions can be "bundled" together to address the overcrowding problem. The bundled solutions may include changes to workflow processes, improving health IT to expedite patient flow, and changing staffing such as increasing custodial staff to turn over rooms faster. The bundling approach is useful because many of the factors influencing overcrowding interact with each other, changing a single factor may not be effective, and any observed differences may be difficult to attribute confidently to a single change. Focusing on process changes and the reallocation of resources is critical given the limited resources of most hospital systems.

## Teamwork

The effective delivery of care in the ED requires that multiple roles work together in a coordinated fashion. Teamwork research focuses on understanding and improving the characteristics of the interactions between individuals that are undertaken to accomplish a shared goal. There is an extensive body of research on the variables that influence team performance.[21,22] Researchers have identified several key variables from the teamwork literature that are specifically relevant to the ED:[23–25]

- *Team leadership*. The leader is critical to promoting teamwork, such as coordination and cooperation among team members.
- *Roles and responsibilities*. Team members must have a clear understanding of their specific roles, but also must have the flexibility to adapt their roles as circumstances change.
- *Shared mental models*. Team members must have a common understanding of the task at hand, the roles of other team members, and the objectives.

- *Feedback*. Effective teams provide feedback to facilitate learning from previous experiences.
- *Communication*. Teams must have open communication.
- *Team affect*. Feelings of trust and confidence are important for high performing teams.

Specific teamwork skills have been shown to be critically important to address a variety of ED challenges, such as the role of communication in handoffs[26-29] as there is clearly a relationship between effective teamwork and improved patient safety in health care.[30] The importance of teamwork has prompted a focus on team training using both didactic and simulation-based methods. Formal didactic training has been shown to improve the quality of team behaviors, reduce clinical error rates, and reinforce positive attitudes toward teamwork.[31] Using simulation as a training tool to improve teamwork skills may be particularly effective, and it has been shown that simulation-based training can improve team processes, behaviors, and attitudes.[32-34] Further, the participants in the training find simulation to be a useful method for improving team performance.[33]

## Interruptions

The deleterious effects of interruptions, such as increased task performance time and increased likelihood of error, have been studied extensively in the basic human factors literature and have been acknowledged as a serious problem in health care by both the Institute of Medicine and Agency for Healthcare Research and Quality.[35-41] An interruption is generally defined as an event that diverts the attention of the individual from the task at hand.[42,43] ED providers are particularly susceptible to a large number of interruptions given the unpredictable nature of patient visits and changing patient demands.[44] Interruptions can lead to delays in delivering care, forgetting to complete particular tasks altogether, as well as increased stress and fatigue of the clinician.[43,45-50]

Researchers examining interruptions in the ED have conducted observational studies on clinician workflow and communication patterns to determine the frequency and source of interruptions.[51,52] Studies have shown that emergency physicians are interrupted frequently, with documented rates ranging from 6.6 to 16 interruptions per hour.[43,49,53,54] As the number of patients being managed simultaneously by an emergency physician increases, so do the number of interruptions.[49] Once an emergency physician is interrupted, the physician will only return to the original task 82% of the time. However, the reason for failing to return to the task is unclear.[55] Emergency nurses are interrupted as frequently as 11 times per hour.[55]

Emergency physicians were interrupted most frequently (40%) during documentation-related tasks.[56] Direct care-related tasks, such as patient communication, were interrupted 20% of the time. Physicians were interrupted during professional communication tasks such as meetings with other health care professionals only 5% of the time. With an understanding of the frequency and type of interruptions in the ED the next step is to develop methods for reducing interruptions, and develop strategies for clinicians to improve their management of the interruption-laden environment.

Interruptions do not always have a negative impact on safety as one observational study actually showed that a large percentage of interruptions were deemed to improve the safety of care.[57] Although this area is relatively understudied, this finding suggests that certain interruptions could be part of a resilient system that keeps patients safe in the ED.

## Health IT

As the adoption of electronic health records (EHRs) spreads across health care, the effects on workflow and safety are acutely felt in the time-sensitive environment of the ED. Although health IT applications encompass a broad category, including medical devices like physiologic monitors, this section focuses on the use of EDIS, computerized physician order entry (CPOE) systems, and EHRs.

The patient tracking board, a component of the EDIS, is the electronic analogue of the "dry-erase whiteboard." Both electronic and whiteboard patient trackers organize patients' demographic, location, and clinical information and serve as a primary means of communication among ED staff members. However, the historical evolution of whiteboards differs significantly from that of the EDIS because the whiteboard framework is a true cognitive artifact of work, developed by the frontline workers to support and organize their own work. Whiteboards were also iteratively designed, with changes to the structure (columns, symbols, and functions) performed with the ease of an eraser, straight edge, and a marker. Because of these factors, whiteboards have naturally adapted to support the cognitive work of the local end-users, while EDIS have instead been developed remotely, and may require some users to adapt their workflow to the IT system.[58-60] Some EDIS are more successful than others at supporting the providers' workflow and cognition. There are some clear benefits to EDIS over the traditional whiteboard such as shared access from many locations. However, an overall positive impact on ED functioning as a result of the introduction of an EDIS has yet to be demonstrated, and this may well be due to the difference in the historical evolution of electronic EDIS compared with traditional whiteboards.[61]

Other health IT elements that are critical to the work process in the ED include CPOE and EHRs. These systems can have a dramatic impact on efficiency in the ED as they might shift the order entry role away from administrative support workers to frontline clinical care providers.

This shift creates the potential to both increase and decrease safety.[62,63] An opportunity for error that is inadvertently increased by the introduction of health IT is the selection of the wrong patient. In paper charts, the records of different patients may vary in thicknesses and are placed in different physical locations so that there are visual cues to alert the provider when the wrong chart has been selected. In most health IT systems, however, screens look identical once a patient has been selected, and this can reduce the opportunity for error identification and recovery. Eye tracking studies have shown that a minority of medical providers in the ED verify patient identification information in a CPOE system after selecting a patient.[64]

The use of additional human factors methods, such as proactive risk assessment, have also been documented to help identify hazards before implementation of CPOE systems in other settings, such as the ICU.[65] Other hospital-wide technologies, such as Bar Coding Management Systems have also been investigated in the health care setting with mixed results and acceptance by staff.[66–68]

## Clinical decision-making

Clinical decision-making in the ED has received attention from human factors researchers because emergency physicians treat many undifferentiated patients, who present with a chief complaint, not a diagnosis. This may result in diagnostic errors, which can be attributed to cognitive factors such as memory and reasoning.[69] Conditions in the emergency care environment (such as high stress, time pressure, interruptions, limited patient histories, and uncertainty) create a challenging decision-making environment. Naturalistic decision-making (NDM), a specific method for studying the decision-making process, is a popular method among human factors researchers that helps gain an understanding of how decisions are made in environments where several constraints exist.[70] Using a NDM approach, researchers have studied the numerous cognitive "short-cuts" or decision-making strategies that physicians use.[71,72] Decision-making strategies are useful to address the challenges that are faced in the ED, but some of these strategies contain certain biases that can lead to diagnostic errors, and whose recognition is important to preventing errors.[73] For example, the availability bias occurs when things that readily come to mind are thought to be more frequent. Thus, recent experience may influence a diagnosis and lead to a diagnostic error. These biases are called cognitive dispositions to respond (CDR) and several different CDRs have been described.[73,74] For example, an emergency physician may elect to give heart rate controlling medications to a patient in rapid atrial fibrillation and fail to identify the precipitating condition, such as severe anemia or pulmonary embolus.

More recently, researchers have focused on leveraging technology to facilitate clinical decision-making. The EDIS provides the necessary information to facilitate decision-making in a timely fashion; however, for these systems to be effective, human factors principles must be respected to ensure the information is presented effectively and that the EDIS fits the user's workflow.[74] More advanced clinical decision support systems (CDSS) may detect possible anomalies or interactions that may be problematic given patient data and provide suggested treatments.[75] For example, CDSS may provide a recommendation as to the appropriate dosage of a medication. Studies examining physician performance and patient outcomes with the CDSS suggest that the systems may be effective for drug dosage recommendations and preventive care, but may not be as effective for diagnosis.[76]

## Application to frontline health care workers

At the foundation of human factors is the understanding that humans have certain capabilities (and limitations) that must be taken into consideration when designing a system or system component. Poorly designed processes, interfaces, tools, and systems that place a physical or cognitive burden on the user should be examined to determine how those artifacts can be changed. Training a user to work with a poorly designed system is not an optimal solution. Rather, identifying the problematic aspects of the system and making deliberate changes to the system is the process by which improvements can be made both effective and sustainable.

## Conclusions

Human factors engineers focus on understanding the user's capabilities and applying this knowledge to improve the tools, machines, and systems with which the user interacts. Researchers applying human factors principles to the ED seek to improve efficiency and patient safety. The review of topics provided here highlights several important issues that should be considered by health care workers, leaders, and researchers to advance patient safety using the application of human factors principles in the ED.

As is evident from the review of each topic, the application of human factors principles to the ED is in its infancy and much of the research has been focused on discovering the "nature" of the problem. For example, research on interruptions has focused on quantifying the type of interruptions that occur in the ED to better understand the frequency and source of interruptions. While this is clearly a necessary first step in applying human factors principles in the analysis of processes in the ED, considerable work is needed to transition into developing and testing specific methods of reducing hazards in the ED and improving patient safety.

Through a combination of observational and task analysis, along with testing and training via medical simulation, human factors engineering is a strong tool to improve emergency medicine, in much the same way as it has in other high stakes industries.

## References

1  Salvendy G. (ed.) Handbook of Human Factors and Ergonomics, 4th edn. Hoboken, NJ: John Wiley & Sons, 2012.
2  Kleiner BM. Sociotechnical systems in health care. In: Carayon, P. (ed.) Handbook of Human Factors and Ergonomics in Health Care and Patient Safety. Mahwah: NJ, Lawrence Erlbaum Associates, 2007: pp.79–95.
3  Kirwan B, Ainsworth LK. (eds.) A Guide to Task Analysis. London: Taylor and Francis, 1992.
4  Annett J. Hierarchical task analysis. In: Diaper D, Stanton N. (eds.) Handbook of Cognitive Task Design. Lawrence Erlbaum Assoc. Inc., 2003: pp.67–82.
5  Carayon P, Schoofs Hundt A, Karsh BT, et al. Work system design for patient safety: the SEIPS model. Qual Saf Health Care. 2006;15(Suppl. 1):i50–8.
6  Carayon P, Cartmill R, Hoonakker P, et al. Human factors analysis of workflow in health information technology implementation. In: Carayon P. (ed.) Handbook of Human Factors and Ergonomics in Health Care and Patient Safety, 2nd edn. Boca Raton, FL: Taylor & Francis, 2012: pp.507–19.
7  Baumlin KM, Shapiro JS, Weiner C, Gottlieb B, Chawla N, Richardson LD. Clinical information system and process redesign improves emergency department efficiency. Jt Comm J Qual Patient Saf. 2010;36(4):179–85.
8  Holden RJ. Lean thinking in emergency departments: a critical review. Ann Emerg Med. 2010;56(5):265–78.
9  Clarke DM. Human redundancy in complex, hazardous systems: a theoretical framework. Saf Sci. 2005;43(9):655–77.
10  Roth EM. Uncovering the requirements of cognitive work. Hum Factors. 2008;50(3):475–80.
11  Bleetman A, Sanusi S, Dale T, Brace S. Human factors and error prevention in emergency medicine. Emerg Med J. 2012;29(5):389–93.
12  Wears RL, Perry SJ. Human factors and ergonomics in the emergency department. Ann Emerg Med. 2002;40(2):206–212.
13  Hakimzada AF, Green RA, Sayan OR, Zhang J, Patel VL. The nature and occurrence of registration errors in the emergency department. Int J Med Inform. 2008;77(3):169–75.
14  Jack BW, Chetty VK, Anthony D, et al. A reengineered hospital discharge program to decrease rehospitalization. Ann Intern Med. 2009;150(3):178.
15  Weir CR, Hammond KW, Embi PJ, Efthimiadis EN, Thielke SM, Hedeen AN. An exploration of the impact of computerized patient documentation on clinical collaboration. Int J Med Inform. 2011;80(8):e62–71.
16  Asaro PV, Boxerman SB. Effects of computerized provider order entry and nursing documentation on workflow. Acad Emerg Med. 2008;15(10):908–15.
17  Bernstein SL, Aronsky D, Duseja R, et al. The effect of emergency department crowding on clinically oriented outcomes. Acad Emerg Med. 2009;16(1):1–10.

18 Trzeciak S, Rivers EP. Emergency department overcrowding in the United. Emerg Med J. 2003;20(5):402–5.

19 Schafermeyer RW, Asplin BR. Hospital and emergency department crowding in the United States. Emerg Med. 2003;15(1):22–7.

20 Richardson DB, Mountain D. Myths versus facts in emergency department overcrowding and hospital access block. Med J Aust. 2009;190(7):369–74.

21 Salas E, Stagl KC, Burke CS. 25 years of team effectiveness in organizations: research themes and emerging needs. In: Cooper CL, Robertson IT. (eds.) International Review of Industrial and Organizational Psychology, 19th ed. West Sussex: Wiley, 2004: pp.47–91.

22 Ilgen DR, Hollenbeck JR, Johnson M, Jundt D. Teams in organizations: from input-process-output models to IMOI models. Annu Rev Psychol. 2005;56:517–43.

23 Eppich WJ, Brannen M, Hunt EA. Team training: implications for emergency and critical care pediatrics. Curr Opin Pediatr. 2008;20(3):255–60.

24 Salas E, Rosen MA, King H. Managing teams managing crises: principles of teamwork to improve patient safety in the emergency room and beyond. Theor Issues Ergon Sci. 2007;8(5):381–94.

25 Cole E, Crichton N. The culture of a trauma team in relation to human factors. J Clin Nurs. 2006;15:1257–66.

26 Cheung DS, Kelly JJ, Beach C, et al. Improving handoffs in the emergency department. Ann Emerg Med. 2009;55(2):171–80.

27 Deering S, Johnston LC, Colacchio K. Multidisciplinary teamwork and communication training. Semin Perinatol. 2011;35(2):89–96.

28 Slagle J, Weinger MW, France DJ, et al. Simulation training for rapid assessment and improved teamwork: assessing the impact of a PACU handoff initiative on actual PACU handoffs. Fourteenth International Scientific Symposium on Improving Quality and Value in Health Care, Nashville, TN, December 9, 2008.

29 Hunte GS. Creating safety in an emergency department. Thesis submitted to the University of British Columbia, 2010.

30 Baker DP, Gustafson S, Beaubien J, Salas E, Barach P. Medical teamwork and patient safety: the evidence-based relation. Washington, DC: American Institutes for Research, 2003.

31 Morey JC, Simon R, Jay GD, et al. Error reduction and performance improvement in the emergency department through formal teamwork training: evaluation results of the MedTeams project. Health Serv Res. 2002;37(6):1553–81.

32 Shapiro MJ, Morey JC, Small SD, et al. Simulation based teamwork training for emergency department staff: does it improve clinical team performance when added to an existing didactic teamwork curriculum? Qual Saf Health Care. 2004;13(6):417–21.

33 Small SD, Wuerz RC, Simon R, Shapiro N, Conn A, Setnik G. Demonstration of high-fidelity simulation team training for emergency medicine. Acad Emerg Med. 1999;6(4):312–23.

34 Wallin CJ, Meurling L, Hedman L, Hedegard J, Fellander-Tsai L. Target-focused medical emergency team training using a human patient simulator: effects on behavior and attitude. Med Educ. 2007;41:173–80.

35 Li SYW, Blandford A, Cairns P, Young RM. The effect of interruptions on postcompletion and other procedural errors: an account based on the activation-based goal memory model. J Exp Psychol Appl. 2008;14(4):314–28.

36 Ratwani RM, Trafton JG. A generalized model for predicting postcompletion errors. Top Cogn Sci. 2010;2(1):154–67.

37 Trafton GJ, Monk CA. Task interruptions. Rev Human Factors Ergonom. 2007;3(1):111–126.

38 Hodgetts HM, Jones DM. Interruptions in the Tower of London task: can preparation minimise disruption? Proceedings of the Human Factors and Ergonomics Society 47th Annual Meeting, 2003: pp.1000–4.

39 Eyrolle H, Cellier JM. The effects of interruptions in work activity: field and laboratory results. Appl Ergon. 2000;31(5):537–43.

40 Kohn LT, Corrigan JM, Donaldson MS. (eds). To Err is Human: Building a Safer Health System. Washington, DC: National Academy Press, 2000: p.287.

41 Hickam D, Severance S, Feldstein A, et al. The effect of health care working conditions on patient safety. Agency Healthcare Res Qual. 2003;74:212.

42 Chisholm CD, Dornfeld AM, Nelson DR, Cordell WH. Work interrupted: a comparison of workplace interruptions in emergency departments and primary care offices. Ann Emerg Med. 2001;38(2):146–51.

43 Grundgeiger T, Sanderson P. Interruptions in healthcare: theoretical views. Int J Med Inform. 2009;78(5):293–307.

44 Chisholm CD, Collison BA, Nelson DR, Cordell WH. Emergency department workplace interruptions: are emergency physicians "'interrupt-driven'" and "'multitasking'"? Acad Emerg Med. 2000;7(11):1239–43.

45 Westbrook JI, Coiera E, Dunsmuir WTM, et al. The impact of interruptions on clinical task completion. Qual Saf Health Care. 2010;19(4):284–9.

46 Alvarez G, Coiera E. Interruptive communication patterns in the intensive care unit ward round. Int J Med Inform. 2005;74(10):791–6.

47 Coiera E. The science of interruption. BMJ Qual Saf. 2012;21(5):357–60.

48 Stephens RJ, Fairbanks RJ. Humans and multitask performance: let's give credit where credit is due. Soc Acad Emerg Med. 2012;19(2):3.

49 Chisholm CD, Pencek AM, Cordell WH, Nelson DR. Interruptions and task performance in emergency departments compared with primary care offices. Acad Emerg Med. 1998;5(5):470.

50 Chisholm CD, Weaver CS, Whenmouth LF, Giles B, Brizendine EJ. A comparison of observed versus documented physician assessment and treatment of Pain: the physician record does not reflect the reality. Ann Emerg Med. 2008.

51 Fairbanks RJ, Bisantz AM, Sunm M. Emergency department communication links and patterns. Ann Emerg Med. 2007;50(4):396–406.

52 Hollingsworth JC, Chisholm CD, Giles BK, Cordell WH, Nelson DR. How do physicians and nurses spend their time in the emergency department? Ann Emerg Med. 1998;31(1):87–91.

53 Laxmisan A, Hakimzada F, Sayan OR, Green RA, Zhang J, Patel VL. The multitasking clinician: decision-making and cognitive demand during and after team handoffs in emergency care. Int J Med Inform. 2006;76(11–12);801–11.

54 Westbrook JI, Coiera E, Dunsmuir WT, et al. The impact of interruptions on clinical task completion. Qual Saf Health Care. 2010;

55 Brixey JJ, Tang Z, Robinson DJ, et al. Interruptions in a level one trauma center: a case study. Int J Med Inform. 2008;77(4):235–41.

56 Brixey JJ, Robinson DJ, Johnson CW, et al. Towards a hybrid method to categorize interruptions and activities in healthcare. Int J Med Inform. 2006;76(11–12):812–20.

57 Walders KC, DiFonzo N. The effect of interruptions on prospective memory in the emergency department. Department of Psychology MS, 2012: pp.1–62.

58 Pennathur P, Cao D, Bisantz AM, et al. Emergency department patient-tracking system evaluation. Int J Ind Ergon. 2011;41:360–9.

59 Bisantz AM, Pennathur PR, Fairbanks RJ, et al. Emergency department status boards: a case study in information systems transition. J Cogn Eng Decis Making. 2010;4(1):39–68.

60 Wears RL, Perry SJ. Status boards in accident and emergency departments: support for shared cognition. Theor Issues Ergon Sci. 2007;8(5):371–80.

61 Rasmussen R. Electronic whiteboards in emergency medicine: a systematic review. In: The 2nd ACM SIGHIT International Health Informatics Symposium. New York, NY: ACM, 2102: pp.483–92.

62 Han YY, Carcillo JA, Venkataraman ST, et al. Unexpected increased mortality after implementation of a commercially sold computerized physician order entry system. Pediatrics. 2005;116(6):1506–12.

63 Del Beccaro MA, Jeffries HE, Eisenberg MA, Harry ED. Computerized provider order entry implementation: no association with increased mortality rates in an intensive care unit. Pediatrics. 2006;118(1):290–5.

64 Henneman PL, Fisher DL, Henneman EA, et al. Providers do not verify patient identity during computer order entry. Acad Emerg Med. 2008;15:1–8.

65 Hundt AS, Adams JA, Schmid JA, et al. Conducting an efficient proactive risk assessment prior to CPOE implementation in an intensive care unit. Int J Med Inform. 2013;82(1):25–38.

66 Holden RJ, Brown RL, Alper SJ, Scanlon MC, Patel NR, Karsh BT. That's nice, but what does IT do? Evaluating the impact of bar coded medication administration by measuring changes in the process of care. Int J Ind Ergon. 2011;41:370–9.

67 Koppel R, Wetterneck T, Telles JL, Karsh BT. Workarounds to barcode medication administration systems: their occurrences, causes, and threats to patient safety. J Am Med Inform Assoc. 2008;

68 Patterson ES, Cook RI, Render ML. Improving patient safety by identifying side effects from introducing bar coding in medication administration. J Am Med Inform Assoc. 2002;9(5):540–53.

69 Kachalia A, Gandhi TK, Puopolo AL, et al. Missed and delayed diagnoses in the emergency department: a study of closed malpractice claims from 4 liability insurers. Ann Emerg Med. 2007;49(2):196–205.

70 Patel VL, Zhang J, Yoskowitz NA, Green R, Sayan OR. Translational cognition for decision support in critical care environments: a review. J Biomed Inform. 2008;41(3):413–31.

71 Kovacs G, Croskerry P. Clinical decision making: an emergency medicine perspective. Acad Emerg Med. 1999;6(9):947–52.

72 Croskerry P. Achieving quality in clinical decision making: cognitive strategies and detection of bias. Acad Emerg Med. 2002;9(11):1184–204.

73 Croskerry P. The importance of cognitive errors in diagnosis and strategies to minimize them. Acad Med. 2003;78(8):775–80.

74 Taylor TB. Information management in the emergency department. Emerg Med Clin North Am. 2004;22(1):241–57.

75 Hunt DL, Haynes RB, Hanna SE, Smith K. Effects of computer-based clinical decision support systems on physician performance and patient outcomes: a systematic review. J Am Med Assoc. 1998;280(15):1339–46.

## CHAPTER 5

# Information technology in emergency care

**Adam Landman[1,2] and E. Gregory Marchand[3,4]**

[1]Health Information Innovation and Integration Brigham and Women's Hospital, USA
[2]Department of Emergency Medicine, Harvard Medical School, USA
[3]Department of Emergency Medicine, MedStar Washington Hospital Center, USA
[4]MedSTAR Transport Services, USA

The concept of an electronic health record (EHR) has been present since the 1960s. At that time, systems such as Problem Oriented Medical Information Systems (PROMIS) at the University of Vermont, promoted the idea of fast, safe, and efficient patient care due to the ready access to data.[1] In 1998, Smith and Feied[2] predicted the future of emergency medicine and electronic records, envisioning systems that allow seamless access to patient information, regardless of the source. Data would flow to providers and would be easily viewed and acted upon, with no piece of data further away than a few milliseconds or two mouse clicks. Such a system would also be supportive of clinical workflow. They predicted that systems would be fully functional and fully adopted in 10 years. In 2004, Taylor[3] revisited this topic and found that while computing systems had grown exponentially in their power and functionality, the use of them in the emergency department (ED) had not met these predictions. This is largely still the case today.

## Emergency department information system features

An emergency department information system (EDIS) is an EHR system designed specifically to manage data and workflow in support of ED patient care and operations.[4] The EDIS must support key ED tasks

*Emergency Care and The Public's Health*, First Edition.
Edited by Jesse M. Pines, Jameel Abualenain, James Scott and Robert Shesser.
© 2014 John Wiley & Sons, Ltd. Published 2014 by John Wiley & Sons, Ltd.

including tracking patient locations, recording clinical documentation, entering orders and reviewing results, and discharge management. As the ED is essentially a microcosm of the hospital, and for that matter of a healthcare system as a whole, many of these features are similar to the core features of ambulatory and hospital EHR systems. Clinical documentation allows all clinicians to record their notes, usually using a combination of free text description and structured data elements. Computerized provider order entry (CPOE) allows clinicians to order medications as well as laboratory and radiology studies; results can then be viewed electronically. Here, we highlight several unique features of EDIS, including patient tracking, discharge management, and dashboard management.

An essential feature of EDIS is patient tracking or electronic whiteboard, allowing continuous passive monitoring of the patients as they pass through the hospital.[5] The ebb and flow of patients through the ED is random, both in volume and acuity of illness. One of the primary challenges in such an environment is quickly and accurately locating the patient in the department and throughout the hospital. EDIS with patient tracking provides an instant view enabling providers to accurately locate patients minute by minute (Figure 5.1). Some EDIS rely on clinical staff to update patient location manually; other systems use radio-frequency identification (RFID) technology to update the patient's location automatically. The tracking board can also provide information on the patient's status, such

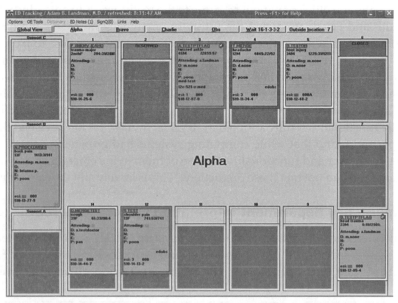

**Figure 5.1** ED tracking system in use at the Brigham and Women's Hospital Emergency Department, Boston, MA.

as waiting to be seen, waiting for test results, needing reassessment, and awaiting discharge. These visual reminders can be helpful communication tools to keep ED flow moving smoothly and efficiently.

EDIS must support the disposition of the patient: discharge home (most common) or admission to the hospital. For treated and discharged patients, EDIS must make it easy for the clinician to provide the patient with accurate and complete discharge instructions, highlighting the patient's diagnosis, care instructions, major procedures/tests performed, follow-up plans, and medication instructions (Figure 5.2). Further, many EDIS also support electronic prescribing where prescriptions are electronically sent to the patient's pharmacy. Well-designed EDIS can enhance the discharge process for both the provider and the patient, by making it easy to provide the patient with high yield discharge instructions.

EDIS must also support patients who are admitted to the hospital. The EDIS should be integrated with the hospital's bed management system, allowing bidirectional communication between the systems. ED providers can then enter an admission order or bed request into EDIS and this will be transferred to the hospital's bed management system and processed by the admitting department (Figure 5.3). When a bed is available, the bed management system will then communicate with the EDIS and notify the ED providers.

The EDIS also has the ability to provide a snapshot dashboard or operational summary of the ED. For example, with a quick glance the

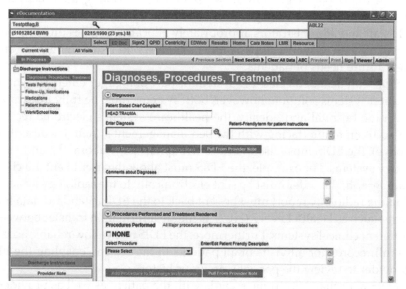

**Figure 5.2** ED electronic discharge instructions module in use at the Brigham and Women's Hospital Emergency Department, Boston, MA.

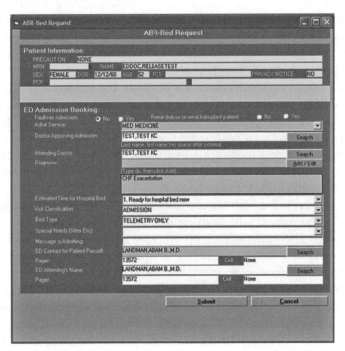

**Figure 5.3** Electronic hospital bed request form in use at the Brigham and Women's Hospital Emergency Department, Boston, MA.

EDIS can inform ED and hospital administrators how many patients are in the department, how many patients are waiting for a bed, and average length of stay (Figure 5.4). This situational awareness can help ED staff and administrators appropriately allocate resources (nursing and ancillary staff as well as inpatient beds) to respond to the immediate and near future needs of patients.

EDIS can be a dedicated ED system or part of a larger enterprise information systems solution; however, both systems must be fully integrated with the hospital and, ideally, the healthcare system's electronic record. In addition to interfacing with the bed management system (as described above), the EDIS must also interface with pharmacy, laboratory, and radiology systems. For example, the EDIS must allow the user to enter a chest radiograph; the order must be sent electronically to the radiology systems and the radiology report must be sent back to the EDIS. Standard data formats, such as Health Level 7 (HL7), facilitate information transfer between different clinical systems. Furthermore, the EDIS must allow reliable access to full records for all visits of all patients to the system, enabling the ED provider to review the patient's previous history.

EDIS may share electronic records with the patient as well as providers beyond the current healthcare organization. Patients are increasingly using personal health records (PHR), secure private electronic applications that

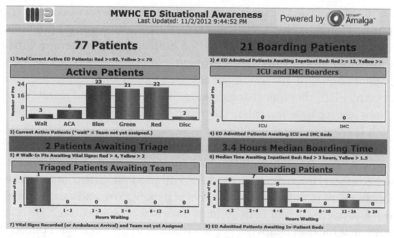

**Figure 5.4** Emergency department situational awareness dashboard from MedStar Washington Hospital Center.

allow patients to access, manage, and share their own health information.[6] Patients can manually update their PHR or the EDIS may be electronically linked to the PHR and automatically update the PHR after the patient's ED visit. EDIS can also facilitate care coordination by electronically sharing ED records with the patient's other healthcare providers. Health information exchange (HIE) provides the capability to share electronic health records across healthcare organizations within a community or region.[7] EDIS supporting HIE can securely share ED visit electronic records with other appropriate healthcare providers, such as the primary care physician who the patient will follow-up with after their ED visit.

## EDIS supports ED workflow

Only meeting functional specifications is inadequate for a useful EDIS. The ideal EDIS must also facilitate the care of ED patients and support clinician's workflow. Consider the case of a 32-year-old female patient presenting to the ED with sharp chest pain, worse with inspiration. The patient currently smokes and is taking oral contraceptives. Commonly, the provider will start the ED visit by interviewing and examining the patient. She will then document the history and physical examination in the EDIS and then review previous electronic records, including past history and medications. The provider will then come up with a differential diagnosis, which would likely include pulmonary embolism. She would then go to the order entry module and place appropriate diagnostic and treatment orders, such as basic labs and a D-dimer. Results of these tests appear in the system when complete; the provider then reviews and documents these findings. The D-Dimer is elevated, so the provider orders a chest computed tomography (CT). In this case, the CT scan confirms pulmonary embolism and the patient is started on anticoagulation therapy. Finally, the provider documents her treatment plan and places an order for inpatient admission for continued anticoagulation and monitoring.

In many EDIS, the clinical documentation, order entry, and results review sections are separate modules. Therefore the provider may be required to switch between several modules or systems to perform key actions, such as reviewing CT scan findings, documenting the results, and ordering the treatment. This typical workflow is disruptive, requiring the provider to move to at least three different modules within a system to complete a task. This can result in delays in care, delays in patient flow, and can potentially cause errors. All current EHR systems have at least some design flaws and require that the user adapt her or his workflow to the system as opposed to the system adapting to the users workflow. One study of the recent adoption of an EHR in a teaching hospital found that workload for residents increased but workload of attending physicians decreased.[8] This changed not only the practice of documenting in the department, but also had an effect on the residents' interactions with the patients, attending physicians, and nurses. In another study, it was noted that while the implementation of an EDIS improved physician satisfaction because of better access to data, the system was also negatively received as a result of the increased demands required to use the documentation system.[9]

In an ideal EDIS, the system supports the clinician's workflow, providing expert decision support and order entry capability while the provider is documenting the history and plan of care. Nursing documentation can be easily reviewed and incorporated into the physician documentation. In the above case, as the provider is recording the complaint of pleuritic chest pain on a wireless device (such as a tablet computer), the nursing electronic documentation noting that the patient is a smoker who takes oral contraceptives is available for the physician to review and include in their social history and medications sections, respectively. The system recognizes the chief complaint of pleuritic chest pain combined with the history of smoking and oral contraceptive use and suggests tests for possible pulmonary embolism. The provider may accept these suggestions and place the orders (or reject these and order different tests) as she completes her assessment and plan. Instead of requiring the provider to look up the test results in a separate module, the EDIS could display the results within the EDIS documentation and allow review and interpretation. Finally, the system could recognize the diagnosis of pulmonary embolism and suggest evidence-based treatment recommendations. This all occurs within the EDIS that the physician is using at the bedside, as she is talking with the patient. This true workflow supportive electronic documentation with integrated CPOE and decision support is still difficult to find in most EDIS.

## Value of EDIS

When implemented properly, EDIS can improve patient safety and provide cost savings by encouraging appropriate and efficient patient care. CPOE of medications has been shown to reduce medication errors, reduce ED length of stay for discharged patients, and reduce time delays in thrombolytic treatment for acute stroke.[10–12] CPOE with decision support has also been shown to improve adherence to treatment guidelines, such as sexual assault prophylaxis recommendations.[13] Sharing and reviewing clinical data through HIE has been shown to improve the cost and efficiency of ED care by reducing hospital admissions as well as radiology and laboratory ordering.[14–16] Further, sharing ED data with public health agencies can automate mandatory disease reporting and also help detect and respond to disease outbreaks.[17] These benefits must be balanced by the potential of EHRs to cause patient harm.[18,19] EDIS must therefore be continuously monitored; safety issues must be reported and addressed in a timely fashion.[20]

## EDIS adoption

Despite the potential for EDIS to improve the quality, efficiency, and safety of ED care, adoption of EDIS has been slow and incomplete. In 2006, less than 2% of US EDs had fully functional EDIS with CPOE, electronic transmission of orders, transmission of public health notifications, and basic decision support capabilities.[21] Just over 10% of US EDs had basic EDIS with CPOE, electronic test results, and electronic clinical documentation. EDs in urban areas were more likely to have basic or fully functional EDIS. While low, these adoption statistics were similar to the adoption rates for basic EHR systems in hospitals (10%) and ambulatory practices (17%) during the same time period.[22,23] In more recent years, adoption of EDIS as well as ambulatory and hospital EHR systems has become much more common as federal policy has helped overcome barriers to adoption.[24–26]

## Barriers to EDIS adoption

A 2006 Robert Wood Johnson Foundation report on the adoption of health information technology (HIT) described four key factors that influence HIT adoption and help explain these low adoption rates:
1 Financial incentives;
2 State of technology;
3 Organizational influences; and
4 Legal and regulatory issues.[27]
We focus the following discussion on how the first three factors are central to EDIS adoption.

In the traditional fee-for-service reimbursement system, there is little financial reward for making large investments in HIT. Hiring more clinicians or purchasing new diagnostic tools has a greater immediate return on investment. Providers generate more charges and receive more reimbursement for seeing more patients, ordering more tests, and performing more procedures. Further, although many studies have shown the value of HIT systems, many physicians and hospital administrators question the value of HIT, citing examples of such systems that reduce efficiency and lead to patient safety concerns.[18,19,28,29] Many health care practices are struggling to meet basic operating expenses and simply do not have funds to invest in technology, training, and support of HIT systems.

The underlying technical design of the HIT system may limit adoption, especially slow or difficult to use systems. The ED is a fast-paced environment; information systems need to be optimized to work in this environment. The system must respond instantaneously; system delays of even a few seconds can be significant in an environment with fast and frequent patient turnarounds. Increased attention is being devoted to the "usability" of information systems, but there are still large opportunities for usability and workflow optimization.[30,31] There are legitimate concerns that EDIS will reduce efficiency; however, evidence from one academic center suggests implementation of EDIS coupled with process redesign can improve revenues and workflow.[32,33] Further, the EDIS must be intuitive and easy to use. Complicated systems increase the risk of errors and can be difficult for new staff to learn. In one case, physicians at Cedars-Sinai Medical Center, Los Angeles, rejected a new CPOE system because it was too difficult to use.[34] Further, some practices are hesitant to invest in high cost technology that may quickly become obsolete.

Characteristics of the organization may also influence EDIS adoption. EDs in urban settings are more likely to adopt basic and fully functional EDIS.[21] Similarly, Jha et al. found that large hospitals, those located in urban areas, and teaching hospitals were more likely to have electronic record systems.[23] EDIS adoption can be more complicated because ED groups may not have direct control over the selection and implementation of the EDIS; the hospital may make these decisions. Ideally, ED leadership maintains close relationships with the hospital and is intimately involved in the selection and implementation of the EDIS. Many of these decisions may be dependent on the organizational leadership and the relationships of the ED group and the hospital. Some leaders will realize the value of EDIS and HIT and lay out a clear plan for adoption; others may not prioritize EDIS adoption. Finally, the culture of the organization can influence the success of adoption and implementation.[35] Many ED staff may be resistant to change (and possibly tired of constant change). Cultivating a culture where HIT is embraced, where staff feel they own the product and are intimately involved in the planning, implementation, and subsequent optimization of the system, may improve the chance of successful system adoption and implementation.

## United States HIT policy: meaningful use

As part of the 2009 American Recovery and Reinvestment Act (ARRA), Congress allocated approximately $27 billion to help overcome financial barriers to HIT adoption and to help ensure HIT was used to improve the quality and efficiency of care and to improve population health.[36,37] The legislation included three components:

1 Establishing the Office of the National Coordinator for Health Information Technology (ONC);

2 Providing financial incentives to providers and hospitals; and

3 Providing additional funding for HIT support activities and tools.

While ONC was already established within the US Department of Health and Human Services, this legislation formalized the office and provided authority and substantial resources to achieve its mission. The majority of the funding was allocated for incentive payments to hospitals and physician offices for adopting and using EHRs. Providers had the potential to receive up to $44,000 over 5 years if implemented in 2011; hospitals could earn several million dollars in incentive payments. Financial penalties imposed on providers and hospitals not meeting requirements by 2015 may further galvanize EHR adoption. For example, eligible providers who do not meet meaningful use criteria by 2015 will lose 1% of their Medicare fees. The legislation also provided funding for health information exchange as well as additional resources to establish support systems and tools for HIT adoption, such as training HIT professionals and establishing regional support centers.

In order to help ensure that HIT funds would improve care, Congress required that hospitals meet meaningful use requirements to qualify for incentive payments.[38] Specifically, meaningful use was designed to improve the quality, safety, efficiency, and reduce health disparities; engage patients and families in their healthcare; improve care coordination; improve population and public health; and preserve the privacy and security of patient's health information. Meaningful use included three components:

1 Using certified EHR products;

2 Using products to perform key tasks (e.g. e-prescribing and electronic exchange of health information); and

3 Capturing and reporting clinical quality measures electronically.

**Table 5.1** Stage 1: Hospital core objectives.[36]

| Core | Objective | Measure |
|------|-----------|---------|
| 1 | CPOE | More than 30% of unique patients with at least one medication in their medication list have at least one medication entered using CPOE |
| 2 | Drug–drug and drug–allergy interaction checks | Functionality must be enabled for the entire EHR reporting period |
| 3 | Record demographics | More than 50% of all unique patients have demographics recorded as structured data |
| 4 | Implement one clinical decision support rule | Implement one clinical decision support rule |
| 5 | Maintain up-to-date problem list of current and active diagnoses | More than 80% of all unique patients seen have at least one entry or an indication that no problems are known for the patient recorded as structured data |
| 6 | Maintain active medication list | More than 80% of all unique patents seen have at least one entry (or an indication that the patient is not currently prescribed any medication) recorded as structured data |
| 7 | Maintain active medication allergy list | More than 80% of all unique patents seen have at least one entry (or an indication that the patient has no known medication allergies) recorded as structured data |
| 8 | Record and chart changes in vital signs | For more than 50% of all unique patients age 2 and over, height, weight, and blood pressure are recorded as structured data |
| 9 | Record smoking status for patients 13 years or older | More than 50% of all unique patients 13 years or older have smoking status recorded as structured data |
| 10 | Report hospital clinical quality measures to CMS or States | For 2011, provide aggregate numerator, denominator, and exclusions through attestation. For 2012, electronically submit clinical quality measures |
| 11 | Provide patients with an electronic copy of their health information, upon request | More than 50% of all unique patients who request an electronic copy of their health information are provided it within 3 business days |
| 12 | Provide patients with an electronic copy of their discharge instructions at time of discharge, upon request | More than 50% of all patients who are discharged who request an electronic copy of their discharge instructions are provided it |
| 13 | Capability to exchange key clinical information among providers of care and patient-authorized entities electronically | Performed at least one test of the certified EHR technology's capacity to electronically exchange key clinical information |
| 14 | Protect electronic health information | Conduct or review a security risk analysis per 45 CFR 164.308(a)(1) and implement updates as necessary and correct identified security deficiencies as part of the hospital's risk management process |

**Table 5.2** Hospital menu set objectives (add reference 36)

| Menu | Objective | Measure |
|---|---|---|
| 1 | Drug-formulary checks | Enabled this functionality and has access to at least one internal or external drug formulary for the entire EHR reporting period |
| 2 | Record advanced directives for patients 65 years or older | More than 50% of all unique patients 65 years old or older admitted to the hospital have an indication of an advance directive status recorded |
| 3 | Incorporate clinical lab test results as structured data | More than 40% of all clinical lab test results ordered are incorporated in certified EHR technology as structured data |
| 4 | Generate lists of patients by specific conditions | Generate at least one report listing patients of the eligible hospital with a specific condition |
| 5 | Use certified EHR technology to identify patient-specific education resources and provide to patient, if appropriate | More than 10% of all unique patients seen are provided patient-specific education resources |
| 6 | Medication reconciliation | The hospital performs medication reconciliation for more than 50% of transitions of care in which the patient is admitted to the hospital |
| 7 | Summary of care record for each transition of care/referrals | The hospital who transitions or refers their patient to another setting of care or provider of care provides a summary of care record for more than 50% of transitions of care and referrals |
| 8 | Capability to submit electronic data to immunization registries/systems* | Performed at least one test of the certified EHR technology's capacity to submit electronic data to immunization registries and follow-up submission if the test is successful |
| 9 | Capability to provide electronic submission of reportable lab results to public health agencies* | Performed at least one test of certified EHR technology's capacity to provide submission of reportable lab results to public health agencies and follow-up submission if the test is successful |
| 10 | Capability to provide electronic syndromic surveillance data to public health agencies* | Performed at least one test of certified EHR technology's capacity to provide electronic syndromic surveillance data to public health agencies and follow- up submission if the test is successful |

CMS, Centers for Medicare and Medicaid Services; CPOE, computerized provider order entry; EHR, electronic health record.
*At least one public health objective must be selected.

From the beginning, the program was designed in stages, with additional features and functionality required in subsequent stages. Stage 1 meaningful use was introduced in 2010 and defined requirements for hospitals and physicians to achieve meaningful use and quality for incentive payments.[39] Hospital EHR systems needed to be certified and meet 14 core objectives plus five objectives from the menu set (Tables 5.1 and 5.2).

Table 5.3 Stage 1: Hospital clinical quality measures.[36]

| | |
|---|---|
| 1* | ED throughput – admitted patients median time from ED arrival to ED departure for admitted patients |
| 2* | ED throughput – admitted patients – admission decision time to ED departure time for admitted patients |
| 3 | Ischemic stroke – discharge on antithrombotics |
| 4 | Ischemic stroke – anticoagulation for atrial fibrillation/flutter |
| 5* | Ischemic stroke – thrombolytic therapy for patients arriving within 2 hours of symptom onset |
| 6 | Ischemic or hemorrhagic stroke – antithrombotic therapy by day 2 |
| 7 | Ischemic stroke – discharge on statins |
| 8 | Ischemic or hemorrhagic stroke – stroke education |
| 9 | Ischemic or hemorrhagic stroke – rehabilitation assessment |
| 10 | VTE prophylaxis within 24 hours of arrival |
| 11 | Intensive care unit VTE prophylaxis |
| 12 | Anticoagulation overlap therapy |
| 13 | Platelet monitoring on unfractionated heparin |
| 14 | VTE discharge instructions |
| 15 | Incidence of potentially preventable VTE |

ED, emergency department; VTE, venous thromboembolism.
*Clinical quality measures involving the emergency department.

In addition, hospitals were required to submit data on 15 clinical quality measures (Table 5.3).

Hospital-based eligible professionals, who provide 90% or more services in the hospital inpatient or ED environments, are not eligible for federal incentive payments. As emergency physicians are hospital-based professionals, they are not eligible for direct incentive payments under the meaningful use guidelines. However, hospitals have the option to include patients seen in the ED to fulfill core and menu objectives. Hospitals therefore have an incentive to support EDIS implementation because EDIS features and use can help them meet meaningful use requirements. Further, several clinical quality measures require reporting ED operational and quality metrics (Table 5.3).

Stage 2 meaningful use requirements were released in 2012, and retain a similar structure to Stage 1, with core and menu objectives.[40] Many of the Stage 2 objectives are the same as Stage 1, but the threshold that providers must meet for the objective has been raised.[41] For example, Stage 1 required CPOE for medications for at least 30% of hospitalized patients. In Stage 2, CPOE is required for more than 60% of medications as well as 30% of laboratory and 30% of radiology orders. A few Stage 1 objectives were either combined or eliminated and almost all the Stage 1 menu objectives are now core objectives under Stage 2. Several

**Table 5.4** Stage 2 core and menu objectives.[38]

| Type (Core/Menu) | Objective | Measure |
| --- | --- | --- |
| Core | Patient ability to view online, download and transmit their health information | Provide time online access to health information for patients within 36 hours of hospital discharge for more than 50% of all patients<br>More than 5% of patients discharged from the hospital can view, download, or transmit to a third party their health information |
| Core | Automatically track medications from order to administration using assistive technologies in conjunction with an e-MAR | All doses of medication are tracked by e-MAR for more than 10% of medication orders |
| Menu | Record electronic notes | Enter at least one electronic progress note for more than 30% of unique patients admitted to the hospital |
| Menu | Electronic imaging results | More than 10% of all scans and tests ordered by a hospital provider that result in an image have the image itself and any explanation or other accompanying information incorporated into or accessible through Certified EHR Technology |
| Menu | Record family history | More than 20% of all unique patients have a structured data entry for one or more first-degree relatives or an indication that family health history has been reviewed |
| Menu | Electronic prescription generation and transmission | More than 10% of hospital discharge medications (for permissible prescriptions) are compared with at least one drug formulary and transmitted electronically using Certified EHR Technology |
| Menu | Structured electronic lab results | Hospital labs send structured electronic clinical lab results to the ordering (ambulatory) provider for more than 20% of electronic lab orders |

EHR, electronic health record; e-MAR, electronic medication administration record.

new objectives were introduced for Stage 2, including use of electronic medication administration and reconciliation (e-MAR) and providing patients the ability to view, download, or access their health information (Table 5.4).[40] Stage 3 meaningful use criteria have been proposed and are under review.[42]

## Conclusions

The 2009 ARRA has increased EHR adoption and use of core EHR features. Unique EDIS features, such as patient tracking, dashboard monitoring, and hospital bed management, may not be specifically incentivized by the ARRA, but should be incorporated into EDIS. Further, vendors should create usable systems that allow providers to work efficiently in high acuity, rapid turnover ED settings. Once core hospital EHR and EDIS features are established, innovative decision support, syndromic surveillance, public health reporting, and other sophisticated tools can be added to improve the care of ED patients. Finally, the impact of HIT on the quality, efficiency, and safety of ED patient care must be continuously monitored and assessed.

## References

1 Schultz S. A history of the PROMIS technology: an effective human interface. 1988. Available at: http://www.campwoodsw.com/mentorwizard/PROMIS History.pdf (accessed 28 November 2013).

2 Smith MS, Feied CF. The next-generation emergency department. Ann Emerg Med. 1998;32(1):65–74.

3 Taylor TB. Information management in the emergency department. Emerg Med Clin North Am. 2004;22(1):241–57.

4 Rothenhaus T, Kamens D, Keaton B, et al. (2009) Emergency Department Information Systems: Primer for Emergency Physicians, Nurses, and IT Professionals. American College of Emergency Physicians: Resolution 22(07) Task Force White Paper. Available at: http://apps.acep.org/WorkArea/DownloadAsset.aspx?id=45756 (accessed 20 January 2013).

5 Aronsky D, Jones I, Lanaghan K, Slovis CM. Supporting patient care in the emergency department with a computerized whiteboard system. J Am Med Inform Assoc. 2008;15(2):184–94.

6 Tang PC, Ash JS, Bates DW, Overhage JM, Sands DZ. Personal health records: definitions, benefits, and strategies for overcoming barriers to adoption. J Am Med Inform Assoc. 2006;13(2):121–6.

7 Baumlin KM, Genes N, Landman A, Shapiro JS, Taylor T, Janiak B. Electronic collaboration: using technology to solve old problems of quality care. Acad Emerg Med. 2010;17(12):1312–21.

8 Park SY, Lee SY, Chen Y. The effects of EMR deployment on doctors' work practices: a qualitative study in the emergency department of a teaching hospital. Int J Med Inform. 2012;81(3):204–17.

9 Callen J, Paoloni R, Li J, et al. Perceptions of the effect of information and communication technology on the quality of care delivered in emergency departments: a cross-site qualitative study. Ann Emerg Med. 2012;61(2):131–44.

10 Kaushal R, Shojania KG, Bates DW. Effects of computerized physician order entry and clinical decision support systems on medication safety: a systematic review. Arch Intern Med. 2003;163(12):1409–16.

11 Spalding SC, Mayer PH, Ginde AA, Lowenstein SR, Yaron M. Impact of computerized physician order entry on ED patient length of stay. Am J Emerg Med. 2011;29(2):207–11.

12 Heo JH, Kim YD, Nam HS, et al. A computerized in-hospital alert system for thrombolysis in acute stroke. Stroke. 2010;41(9):1978–83.

13 Britton DJ, Bloch RB, Strout TD, Baumann MR. Impact of a computerized order set on adherence to centers for disease control guidelines for the treatment of victims of sexual assault. J Emerg Med. 2013;44(2):528–35.

14 Bailey JE, Wan JY, Mabry LM, et al. Does health information exchange reduce unnecessary neuroimaging and improve quality of headache care in the emergency department? J Gen Intern Med. 2013;28(2):176–83.

15 Bailey JE, Pope RA, Elliott EC, Wan JY, Waters TM, Frisse ME. Health information exchange reduces repeated diagnostic imaging for back pain. Ann Emerg Med. 2013;62(1):16–24.

16 Frisse ME, Johnson KB, Nian H, et al. The financial impact of health information exchange on emergency department care. J Am Med Inform Assoc. 2012;19(3):328–33.

17 Shapiro JS, Genes N, Kuperman G, Chason K, Richardson LD, Clinical Advisory Committee H1N1 Working Group NwYCIE. Health information exchange, biosurveillance efforts, and emergency department crowding during the spring 2009 H1N1 outbreak in New York City. Ann Emerg Med. 2010;55(3):274–9.

18 Congressional Budget Office. Evidence on the costs and benefits of health information technology. 2008. Available at: http://www.cbo.gov/sites/default/files/cbofiles/ftpdocs/91xx/doc9168/05-20-healthit.pdf (accessed 28 November 2013).

19 Koppel R, Metlay JP, Cohen A, et al. Role of computerized physician order entry systems in facilitating medication errors. J Am Med Assoc. 2005;293(10):1197–203.

20 Kushniruk AW, Bates DW, Bainbridge M, Househ MS, Borycki EM. National efforts to improve health information system safety in Canada, the United States of America and England. Int J Med Inform. 2013;82(5):e149–60.

21 Landman AB, Bernstein SL, Hsiao AL, Desai RA. Emergency department information system adoption in the United States. Acad Emerg Med. 2010;17(5):536–44.

22 DesRoches CM, Campbell EG, Rao SR, et al. Electronic health records in ambulatory care: a national survey of physicians. N Engl J Med. 2008;359(1):50–60.

23 Jha AK, DesRoches CM, Campbell EG, et al. Use of electronic health records in US hospitals. N Engl J Med. 2009;360(16):1628–38.

24 Selck F, Decker S. Health Information Technology in the Emergency Department. Academy Health Annual Research Meeting 2013; Available at: http://academyhealth.org/files/2013/monday/selck.pdf (accessed 6 December 2013).

25 Hsiao CJ, Jha AK, King J, et al. Office-based physicians are responding to incentives and assistance by adopting and using electronic health records. Health Aff (Millwood). 2013;32(8):1470–7.

26 DesRoches CM, Charles D, Furukawa MF, et al. Adoption of electronic health records grows rapidly, but fewer than half of US hospitals had at least a basic system in 2012. Health Aff (Millwood). 2013;32(8):1478–85.

27 Robert Wood Johnson Foundation. Health Information Technology in the United States: The Information Base for Progress. 2006.

28 Chaudhry B, Wang J, Wu S, et al. Systematic review: impact of health information technology on quality, efficiency, and costs of medical care. Ann Intern Med. 2006;144(10):742–52.

29 Buntin MB, Burke MF, Hoaglin MC, Blumenthal D. The benefits of health information technology: a review of the recent literature shows predominantly positive results. Health Aff (Millwood). 2011;30(3):464–71.

30 Schumacher R, Lowry S. NIST Guide to the Processes Approach for Improving the Usability of Electronic Health Records. 2010.

31 Armijo D, McDonnell C, Werner K. Electronic Health Record Usability: Interface Design Considerations. Agency for Healthcare Research and Quality, 2009.

32 Baumlin KM, Shapiro JS, Weiner C, Gottlieb B, Chawla N, Richardson LD. Clinical information system and process redesign improves emergency department efficiency. Jt Comm J Qual Patient Saf. 2010;36(4):179–85.

33 Shapiro JS, Baumlin KM, Chawla N, et al. Emergency department information system implementation and process redesign result in rapid and sustained financial enhancement at a large academic center. Acad Emerg Med. 2010;17(5):527–35.

34 Benko L. Back to the drawing board; Cedars-Sinai's physician order-entry system suspended. Mod Healthcare. 2003;33(4):12.

35 Van Der Meijden MJ, Tange HJ, Troost J, Hasman A. Determinants of success of inpatient clinical information systems: a literature review. J Am Med Inform Assoc. 2003;10(3):235–43.

36 Blumenthal D. Stimulating the adoption of health information technology. N Engl J Med. 2009;360(15):1477–9.

37 American Recovery and Reinvestment Act of 2009. H.R.1. Available at: http://www.opencongress.org/bill/111-h1/show (accessed 28 November 2013).

38 Blumenthal D, Tavenner M. The "meaningful use" regulation for electronic health records. N Engl J Med. 2010;363(6):501–4.

39 Centers for Medicare and Medicaid Services. Medicare and Medicaid EHR Incentive Program: Meaningful Use Stage 1 Requirements Overview. 2010. Available at: http://www.cms.gov/Regulations-and-Guidance/Legislation/EHRIncentive Programs/downloads/MU_Stage1_ReqOverview.pdf (accessed 28 November 2013).

40 Centers for Medicare and Medicaid Services. Stage 2 Overview Tipsheet. 2012. Available at: http://www.cms.gov/Regulations-and-Guidance/Legislation/EHR IncentivePrograms/Downloads/Stage2Overview_Tipsheet.pdf (accessed 28 November 2013).

41 Centers for Medicare and Medicaid Services. Stage 1 vs. Stage 2 Comparison Table for Eligible Hospitals and CAHs. 2012. Available at: http://www.cms.gov /Regulations-and-Guidance/Legislation/EHRIncentivePrograms/Downloads /Stage1vsStage2CompTablesforHospitals.pdf (accessed 28 November 2013).

42 Department of Health and Human Services Office of the National Coordinator for Health Information Technology. Request for Comment Regarding the Stage 3 Definition of Meaningful Use of Electronic Health Records. 2012. Available at: http://www.healthit.gov/sites/default/files/hitpc_stage3_rfc_final.pdf (accessed 28 November 2013).

# CHAPTER 6

# Telehealth and acute care

## Sara Paradise[1], Michael Kee-Ming Shu[1], and Neal Sikka[2]

[1]Emergency Medicine and Health Policy, The George Washington University, USA
[2]Department of Emergency Medicine, The George Washington University, USA

It is important to begin with defining terms under the umbrella of telehealth services to provide clarity for the purposes of policy and application: [1]

- *Telemedicine* is a term specifically referring to real-time (occurring at the moment) clinical services (e.g., video conferencing between a patient at one location and a physician at a separate location).
- *Store and forward* technology is where patient data or digital images are captured, stored, and sent as a file to a clinician who responds with assessment. An example of this would be images of burn wounds sent to a burn specialist, or X-rays that are sent via a mobile phone or other device to a radiologist.
- *Remote patient monitoring* involves transmitting information from sensors and monitoring equipment such as blood pressure monitors and blood glucose meters to an external monitoring center where they can be reviewed by a health care provider.
- *Mobile health*, or m-Health, includes use of mobile smart phones and PDAs for any function related to patient care.

These definitions were further clarified in the Federal Communications Commission (FCC) Broadband Plan in Chapter 10 dedicated to health care (Figure 6.1). These definitions, not before available in a government document, provide a basis for policy and regulatory discussion.

This chapter provides an overview of the application of telemedicine as it is used in acute care settings, providing explanation and real-life examples of use. While acute care is the focus of this chapter, it is important to recognize that telehealth services can also play a significant part in chronic

*Emergency Care and The Public's Health*, First Edition.
Edited by Jesse M. Pines, Jameel Abualenain, James Scott and Robert Shesser.
© 2014 John Wiley & Sons, Ltd. Published 2014 by John Wiley & Sons, Ltd.

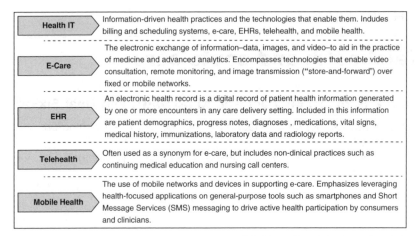

**Figure 6.1** The federal communications commission (FCC) broadband plan broadband plan, chapter 10: Healthcare (http://www.broadband.gov/plan/10-healthcare/).

disease management, as the term "care coordination" closely aligns with use cases of telehealth in part or in the entirety of one's disease process.

## Case study: University of Mississippi Medical Center

The University of Mississippi Medical Center (UMMC) has served as a vanguard for telemedicine since its inception in 2003. With 53 of 82 counties located 40 minutes or more from specialist care, access to quality of care is vital for Mississippi's rural critical access hospitals.[2] "The idea began in 2001. We were getting a lot of frantic phone calls from nurse practitioners all over the state asking for the helicopter to transfer patients. That concerned us," reported Dr Robert Galli, executive director of the TelEmergency Program Professor, and past Chairman of emergency medicine at the UMMC.[3]

UMMC trains and places specially trained nurse practitioners in a variety of rural emergency departments (EDs), where workers serve patients under the clinical supervision of emergency staff via a telemedicine video link – TelEmergency. "Through the screens, we can talk to the patients. They see us and we see them," said Galli.[3] This helps address the inadequate physician and nursing workforce of rural health care providers, minimizing unnecessary travel for healthcare and keeping patients closer to home, family, and work.[4] Galli advocated: "It's basically putting a board certified physician at these tiny rural hospitals with the nurse practitioner being the hands-on technician."[3] Now with over 10 years' experience, a telepsychiatry sector beginning in 2008, and an Office of Telehealth since

2012, the UMMC provides 24/7 telehealth support for physicians, nurses, and technology staff.[2]

Feedback with the TelEmergency pilot program at UMMC yielded remarkable results: 94% of staff reported they were "comfortable or very comfortable with the system." An astounding 98.7% stated that they were able to communicate with the collaborating physician without difficulty. A total of 87.3% believed that their care was as good as or better than they would have received with a physician alone. Furthermore, 91.2% of patients stated that they were likely to return to the facility knowing that the TelEmergency service was available. At the end of the pilot study, seven of eight hospitals surveyed were pleased with the program's results and opted to continue their participation.[4] "We need to get the word out that it is actually working," said Dr Galli.[3]

## ED specialty consultations

ED physicians are masters at multi-tasking and triaging patients. However, some diagnoses have beneficial but risky treatments that are best administered in conjunction with other medical specialists. We examine the role of telemedicine in the management of acute stroke, rapid interpretation of radiologic images, and management of traumatic injury.

### Case study: telestroke

The motto "time equals brain" signifies the importance of acute stroke intervention with t-PA, a thrombolytic agent used for ischemic stroke which has a 4.5-hour window period of administration. The use of t-PA involves a series of complex decision-making processes, often best managed by an experienced provider. One such method to increase the use of t-PA is the adoption of primary stroke centers (PSCs), which must meet criteria of providing 24/7 ability to diagnose and treat patients with stroke, among other strict criteria outlined by the Joint Commission.[5]

Unfortunately, PSCs represent a minority of facilities across the United States. For this reason, it is hoped that the involvement of remote experts in stroke management, termed "telestroke", will bring the highest standard of care to patients in rural, community, and urban centers alike. The system functions with a "hub and spoke" model, where the hub is the PSC with a vascular neurologist available for consultation, and the spokes are non-PSC facilities staffed primarily by emergency physicians.[6]

One such successful program includes Remote Evaluation of Acute Ischemic Stroke (REACH), a low-cost web-based system that provides such a link between the Medical College of Georgia and eight rural community hospitals in east central Georgia. In this model, the vascular neurologist at the hub site logs into the REACH web site to access patients' observations, review CT images via DICOM software, and perform a video consultation over broadband internet to determine a National Institutes of Health Stroke Scale (NIHSS) score and give the appropriate t-PA recommendations. In addition to sparing patient treatment time, the requirements of the "spoke" hospital are feasible: a CT scanner capable of transmitting DICOM imaging, broadband internet access and equipment costs less than $10 000.[7]

It is important to note that PSC-underserved areas exist even in urban environments. This highlights one of the main barriers to telemedicine for stroke in the current model, as reimbursement is only limited to services performed in a "rural health professional shortage area" or in a "county not classified as a metropolitan statistical area."[6] In the future, this loophole must be addressed to allow greater access to stroke consultation.

## Case study: teleradiology

Teleradiology is a branch of telemedicine that has been saturated for well over a decade, providing good hindsight on the rapid change in infrastructure and the aftermath of transitioning from an on-site to remote form of communication. The number of providers utilizing teleradiology jumped from 15% in 2003 to 50% in 2007, and has remained around that level since then.[8] Initially, coverage mostly consisted of "night hawks" covering off-hours shifts. With increasing accessibility to bandwidth, companies providing low-cost interpretations with rapid turnaround time – 30 minutes for preliminary reports and 24 hours for final reports – began to emerge. The Joint Commission began to accredit such companies in 2004, further establishing their place in the world of radiology.[8]

One of the largest providers of teleradiology currently is Minnesota-based VRad, which partnered with NightHawk in 2010 to expand its coverage to over 2700 health care facilities nationwide. According to the CTO Rick Jennings, VRad has spent $50 million over the last 8 years extending its IT infrastructure, stating "we were cloud before it was called the cloud."[9]

While teleradiology is surely an added benefit in emergency situations when indications for studies are limited, limitations in patient care do exist. Coordination of care, such as compiling final reports based on follow-up examinations, imaging study comparisons, and collaborations across specialists, is difficult to achieve. Additionally, several radiologists reviewing a patient's images across time may create incongruence in treatment and care.[8]

## Case study: teletrauma

Eastern Maine Medical Center (EMMC) in Bangor, Maine, is one of the state's three regional trauma centers, serving as the referral center for over 20 community-level hospitals. In 2004, they became the first center to gain telepresence through live audiovisual consultation to 11 sites throughout the state. With initial start-up costs totaling $70,000, maintenance of the system has been facilitated by internet provider-based services, utilizing large video screens that display the trauma bay at remote sites.[10]

Their implementation demonstrates a number of valuable lessons on the impact of teletrauma. By involvement in the initial patient survey, experienced trauma physicians present through telepresence recommend the most current practices in the field. By bypassing obsolete practices such as "spine clearance," advising against computer tomography (CT) scans and X-rays in certain cases, and providing advice on how to manage more stable patient subtleties, such as the current guidelines for reversal of therapeutic anticoagulation, they decrease transfer time while providing optimal patient care.[10] Perhaps one of the most interesting observations through their experience is the enhanced sense of teamwork and partnership amongst those participating in teletrauma interactions, causing them to coin the term "the 130 million square foot trauma room."[10]

A challenging aspect to the teletrauma program at EMMC is that trauma surgeons, while available 24/7, are often not physically at the computer sites that interconnect to the remote hospitals; additionally, there are cumbersome menus to navigate, causing a phone call to suffice in more emergent cases.[10] As with all considerations, financial reimbursement for services is a concern, and will likely drive the expansion or demise of such programs.

## Extending ED provider access

With a relative shortage of emergency physicians compared to the volume of patients seeking care in EDs, providers such as nurse practitioners (NPs) and physician assistants (PAs) have become an increasingly vital part of the ED workforce. While scope of practice varies state-by-state, in general, NPs and PAs have the capacity to make medical decisions under direct supervision of ED physicians.

But what is the scope of their use, and how effective are PAs as a supplement to ED physicians? Data from the National Hospital Ambulatory Medical Care Survey showed that between 1993 and 2009, NPs and PAs serviced approximately 1.8 billion ED visits, with PAs staffing about 6.3% of visits and NPs about 2.5%.[11] Benefits of incorporating NPs and PAs are cost reduction, supplementing provider shortage areas (i.e. rural settings), decreasing emergency room wait times, and helping with transition of care to inpatient settings. Limitations include scope of practice issues in some rural settings, where PAs may serve as the sole practitioner, or limited experience assessing and intervening in more high-acuity situations.

Therefore, the use of NPs and PAs is optimal in a setting where an ED physician is also present, actually or virtually, to provide guidance and professional support, but can definitely provide a high level of care to patients seeking care in both urban and remote emergency settings.[11]

## Nurse advice lines

Nurse advice and designated telephone triage lines have been established for many years, and are one of the most commonly used services; a Swedish study citing millions of calls each year for patients seeking health care advice.[12] The flow of a telephone encounter is that the nurse answers the calls, provides advice, and essentially helps to triage the patient based on their perceived acuity. More than simply answering health questions, phone-based communication is a difficult endeavor, as it requires excellent communication skills to assess the patient's condition, understand their symptoms, and to make an accurate assessment.

In 2005, the Kids Kare Line in Australia conducted a comprehensive evaluation of telephone triage services in which experienced registered nurses responded to parents' requests for health care advice for their child. The study proved that using phone consultations as a telehealth service is a highly effective way to triage and treat patients, vastly reducing costs while greatly increasing medical care quality. Out of 101 parents, all but five reported that they were answered promptly and understood the advice; 96% were satisfied with the advice received. In follow-up, 50 parents identified that they had not used another service or health practitioner for the same issue afterwards.[13] A consolidated and standard practice for nurse advice lines could revolutionize healthcare and bring telemedicine to the forefront of primary care in the future.[12]

## Online medical consultations

For low-acuity visits, online medical consultations using video, telephone, or online messaging have been marketed as delivering quality affordable care while patients are at home or wherever they can find an internet connection. With the adoption of electronic health records (EHR) systems, this functionality has become more feasible, allowing patients and their primary care providers to have an online forum for medical visits. Patients can fill out a questionnaire about symptoms, review their medication list, allergies, and assign a pharmacy such that the physician is able to review and make the appropriate assessment and plan all via an online forum. While this tends to attract a certain demographic of young internet-savvy users, a 2011 study based at the University of Pittsburgh Medical Center found that 88% of patients were satisfied with their e-visit, and of those 99% would complete another e-visit.[13]

Aside from "traditional" primary care e-visits, online medical consulting companies such as American Well and Teledoc have capitalized on this market to provide services independent of any particular clinic or hospital using the patient's own webcam. Teledoc, a Dallas-based telehealth provider established in 2002, offers board-certified internal medicine consultations 24/7, 365 days a year, providing a less-expensive alternative to the ED for non-emergency complaints. "We're a clinical services company using technology to improve access and as a byproduct driving down cost to the healthcare system," said Jason Gorevic, CEO of Teledoc.[14] Similarly, American Well, established in 2006, uses their software program Online Care to enhance the online experience to include live patient–doctor interactions on demand. Convenience is key, with downloadable EHR records, ePrescribing, automatic payment, and apps for iPhone and iPad being their marketable features.[15]

Despite the perceived benefit of avoiding a trip to the doctor's office, these e-visits have been slow to be adopted by the general public. As Roy Schoenberg, the CEO of American Well, argues, the greatest barrier to these services is not reimbursement, but rather the lack of understanding of how telehealth can have a role in today's society.[16] In Australia, for example, the Medicare program is offering 50% bonuses to specialists who adopt telehealth technology and 35% bonuses to doctors, nurses, and midwives who participate in video consultations with patients, according to Healthcare IT news.[17] These adaptations to the current system would likely provide incentive to incorporate their use in a widespread fashion.

## Patient centered triage tools

The most widely used version of telehealth is the internet, where consumers are able to immediately access health information from any internet connection. This trend is confirmed by data from the Health Information National Trends survey in the United States, which showed that 48.6% of patients use the internet as their initial resource for accessing health information, with only 10.9% of US adults going to their physicians.[18]

Physicians can usually easily identify this subset of patients by their abundant use of medical terminology and description of "classic" symptoms related to their "diagnosis." While online access to health information can be beneficial in certain settings, those patients who undergo "cyberchrondria," or internet-guided self-diagnosis, for every ache and pain can prove to be detrimental to the patient and physician alike. Similarly, patients who access information online and downplay their symptoms could set themselves up for complications.[19]

This is especially unsettling considering that a report by Pew Internet and American Life Project stated that 75% of patients do not verify the source and the date of health information found online.[18] Furthermore, a 2011 *New York Times* article titled "Prescription for fear" identified the disparity in search engine quality, stating that "WebMD has become permeated with pseudomedicine and subtle misinformation," due to connections with BigPharma and ad revenues upwards of $500 million in 2010. Contrast this with MayoClinic, a non-profit medical practice and research group, with neatly organized, reliable access to information.[19]

Therefore, it is important that physicians spend time educating patients on reliable sources of information. Standards of searching for online health information by the Joint Commission include details on web sites that provide clinically proven, unbiased, and reliable health care information; explanations and backgrounds on each web site; useful "net-surfing" strategies for finding well-researched health information; and specific health care topics from dozens of trusted information sources. They identify top resources to include healthfinder.gov, www.nlm.nih.gov, and www.mayoclinic.com, noting the absence of more popular sites like WebMD and MedLine.[20]

## Remote patient monitoring and follow-up

Remote patient monitoring includes various methods of evaluating patients from afar. Transmission of patients' observations, laboratory data, and even management of patients at remote sites all are under the spectrum of remote patient monitoring. More recently, these services have been increasingly utilized in response to a nationwide shortage of highly trained critical care specialists in the United States. Thus, intensive care unit (ICU) remote monitoring was designed to help intensivists access clinical data and interact with bedside caregivers from a remote site, promoting continuous and proactive patient management in ICUs. These services have been proven to decrease mortality, incidence of complications, and length of stay, all while considerably reducing ICU costs.[21]

At the University of Texas Health Science Center, Houston, investigations proved the viability of remote patient monitoring utilizing telehealth. With a remote monitoring team consisting of two intensivists, four registered nurses, and two administrative technicians, the team monitors patients at remote sites.[21] Physician roles included direct clinical decisions and patient interventions, attending to patient data presented through the Clinical Information System, and documentation of clinical decision-making.[21]

Concerns regarding the growth of telehealth for use of patient monitoring include interruption of workflow by technology problems, which could prove damaging to a newly implemented system.[21]

A more simplistic value of remote patient monitoring is in the form of text messaging. As a contemporary and cost-effective way to help enhance the continuum of care in a remote monitoring format, the ability to reach the masses affords hospitals the opportunity to send reminders to patients to take their medication, test their blood sugar, and the dates and time of their follow-up appointments.[22] However, providers must be vigilant about Health Insurance Portability and Accountability Act (HIPAA) compliance, as patient identifiers should not be sent over the phone. If the patient's name or ID number containing any results or information is sent, it falls under the rules of HIPAA and is considered a patient health identifier, or ePHI. Complying with HIPAA to send ePHI is cumbersome, as it requires a phone that is locked and secured, with only transmission of encrypted messages through mobile companies that have signed a Business Associate Agreement with the hospital or health care company.[22] Luckily, medical apps developed for this purpose are exceedingly useful in the transmission of texts as a form of remote patient monitoring.

## mHealth

Recently named one of the top health care initiatives by the director of the National Institutes of Health, Francis Collins,[23] an exploding area of telehealth is mobile health or mHealth.[23] An estimated 84% of physicians are already using smartphones (with 25% additionally using tablets) to access more than 13,000 smartphone apps available for medical decision-making.[24] Collins states that mHealth apps are just beginning to transition from "gee-whiz toys" to a low-cost real-time way to assess disease, movement, images, behavior, social interactions, environmental toxins, metabolites, and a host of other physiologic variables. Indeed, video consultations with crystal clear image quality, audio, and video with zoom capacity, mobile phones seem to be a logical way to enhance patient care.[23]

## Medical apps

Similarly, apps have been developed with the intent of allowing patients to check their symptoms and arrive at a diagnosis. One such app is iTriage, a free app created by two ED physicians in 2008 that "helps you answer the questions. What medical condition could I have? Where should I go for treatment? Save, easily access, and share the healthcare information that's most important to you." Acquired by Aetna in 2013, criticism of such apps includes patients being directed to specific "endorsed" EDs.[25]

## Integration with quality drivers

In February 2009, the American Recovery and Reinvestment Act (ARRA) published the Health Information Technology for Economic and Clinical Health (HITECH) provisions, which established financial incentives of up to $44,000 per provider for demonstrating meaningful use of EHRs, and if not met by 2015, financial penalties.[26] This effected a rapid increase in use of EHRs, jumping provider and hospital use from 17% and 8%, respectively, to a goal of over 50% of providers and 80% of hospitals demonstrating meaningful use in 2013.[27]

Much of this was in anticipation of the 2010 passage of the Patient Protection and Affordable Care Act, which focuses on incorporating public health measures into the current health care system. Specifically, the Centers for Medicaid and Medicare Services has begun a quality improvement process that includes quarterly reporting and publication of specific data measures related to diseases such as acute myocardial infarction, heart failure, pneumonia, and surgical care. For example, all patients admitted to the hospital with a diagnosis of congestive heart failure must receive smoking cessation counseling if currently smoking, prescription of an angiotensin-converting enzyme inhibitor or an angiotensin receptor blocker if ejection fraction is less than 40%, and appropriate discharge education and follow-up is established. Additionally, for Medicare patients over 65 years, all-cause mortality and readmission rates are reviewed as part of reimbursement.[28]

These examples present a unique challenge for facilities, as these new guidelines require extensive implication of processes to ensure that measures are being met and financial penalties avoided. Concerns about privacy and security, legal and regulatory barriers, and technical concerns all factor into the implementation of what federal government, patients, and physicians alike hope will provide a better quality, coordinated care system through more robust use of EHRs.[27]

## References

1 American Telemedicine Association website. 2013. Available at: http://www.americantelemed.org/practice/nomenclature (accessed 28 November 2013).
2 University of Mississippi Medical Center. Telehealth. Available at: http://www.umc.edu/telehealth/ (accessed 28 November 2013).

3 Barron M. UMC telemergency program. Available at: http://www.innovate.ms/pointe-innovation/view.php?entryID=2140 (acessed 28 November 2013).

4 Galli R, Keith J, McKenzie K, Hall G, Henderson K. Telemergency: a novel system for delivering emergency care to rural hospitals. Ann Emerg Med. 2008; 51(3):275–84.

5 The Joint Commission. Advanced certification for primary stroke centers. Available at: http://www.jointcommission.org/certification/primary_stroke_centers.aspx (accessed 28 November 2013).

6 Demaerschalk BM, Miley ML,Kiernan TJ, Bobrow BJ, et. al. Stroke telemedicine. Mayo Clin Proc. 2009; 84(1):53–64.

7 Hess D, Wang S, Gross H, Hall C, Adams R. Telestroke: extending stroke expertise into underserved areas. Lancet Neurol 2006; 5:275–8.

8 Steinbrook R. The age of teleradiology. N Engl J Med. 2007; 357(1):5–7.

9 Versel N. VRad extends cloud radiology services. 2011. Available at: http://www.informationweek.com/healthcare/interoperability/vrad-extends-cloud-radiology-services/231601187 (accessed 28 November 2013).

10 Bjorn PR. Rural teletrauma: applications, opportunities, and challenges. Adv Emerg Nurs J. 2012; 34(3):232–7.

11 Brown D, Sullivan A, Espinola J, Camargo C. Continued rise in the use of mid-level providers in us emergency departments, 1993–2009. J Emerg Med. 2012; 5(1):21.

12 Keatinge D,Rawlings K. Outcomes of a nurse-led telephone triage service in Australia. Int J Nurs Pr. 2005; 11(1):5–12.

13 Albert SM, Shevchik GJ, Paone S, Martich DG. Internet-based medical visit and diagnosis for common medical problems: experience of a first-user cohort. Telemed e-Health. 2011; 17(4):304–8.

14 Teladoc. Available at: www.teladoc.com (accessed 28 November 2013).

15 American Well. Available at: http://www.americanwell.com/pressRelease_American_Well_Launches_Industrys_Most_Comprehensive_Infrastructure_for_Telehealth.html (accessed 12 December 2013).

16 Glenn B. The biggest barrier to telemedicine adoption isn't reimbursement. 2012. Available at: http://medcitynews.com/2012/04/the-biggest-barrier-to-telemedicine-adoption-isnt-reimbursement/ (accessed 28 November 2013).

17 Wicklund E. Australian government launches telehealth initiative. 2011. Available at: http://www.healthcareitnews.com/news/australian-government-launches-telehealth-initiative (accessed 28 November 2013).

18 Fox S. Online Health Search 2006. Pew Internet and American Life Project. 2006.

19 Heffernan V. A prescription for fear. The New York Times. 2011.

20 The Joint Commission. How to find reliable health information. Available at: http://www.jointcommission.org/assets/1/18/patient_101.pdf (accessed 28 November 2013).

21 Tang Z, Weavind L, Mazabob J, Thomas E, Chu-Weininger M, Johnson T. Workflow in intensive care unit remote monitoring: a time-and-motion study. Crit Care Med. 2007; 35(9):2507–63.

22 Kangas E. Is text messaging HIPAA compliant? 2012. Available at: http://luxsci.com/blog/is-text-messaging-hipaa-compliant.html (accessed 28 November 2013).

23 Collins F. The real promise of mobile health apps. Sci Am. July 10, 2012.

24 Dolan B. Report: 13K iPhone consumer health apps in 2012. 2011. Available at: http://mobihealthnews.com/13368/report-13k-iphone-consumer-health-apps-in-2012/ (accessed 28 November 2013).

25 itriage health. Available at: https://www.itriagehealth.com/ (accessed 28 November 2013).

26 Adler-Milstein J, DesRoches CM, Jha A. Health information exchange among US hospitals. Am J Manag Care. 2011; 17(11):761–8.

27 US Department of Health and Human Services. Doctors and hospitals' use of health IT more than doubles since 2012. 2013. Available at: http://www.hhs.gov/news/press/2013pres/05/20130522a.html (accessed 28 November 2013).

28 Centers for Medicare and Medicaid Services. National impact assessment of medicare quality measures. 2012. Available at: http://www.cms.gov /Medicare/Quality-Initiatives-Patient-Assessment-Instruments/QualityMeasures /Downloads/NationalImpactAssessmentofQualityMeasuresFINAL.pdf (accessed 12 December 2013).

# CHAPTER 7

# Simulation in emergency care

## Claudia Ranniger[1] and Keith E. Littlewood[2]

[1]Department of Emergency Medicine, USA
[2]School of Medicine, University of Virginia, USA

## Introduction

On-the-job training alone cannot adequately prepare emergency department (ED) providers for the diversity of clinical presentations they are expected to manage. Rare yet emergent procedures, complex patient presentations requiring coordination of multiple care providers, and management decisions in resource-limited situations such as mass casualty events are all tasks in which ED providers are expected to be proficient, yet for which routine clinical practice may not provide adequate training. Simulation – the use of trained actors, anatomic models, computer-based task trainers and mannequins, and virtual reality environments to create realistic care scenarios in a purely educational setting – can provide crucial training in the procedural, communications, and teamwork skills required to provide high-quality medical care. This chapter identifies the performance gaps in clinical training, the learning theories, and evaluation methods that support the efficacy of simulation-based education, and discusses how simulation training is currently being used to address the identified performance gaps in emergency medicine.

## Performance gaps in emergency medicine

Performance gaps can be defined as the difference in the desired patient outcome and the actual outcome that occurs with failure to provide highest quality medical care. Medical errors, estimated to cause up to 98 000 deaths and many more injuries yearly, occur in four domains:[1]
- *Errors of diagnosis* including a wrong diagnosis or a delay in diagnosis;
- *Errors in treatment* including incorrect performance of a procedure or a medication mishap;

*Emergency Care and The Public's Health*, First Edition.
Edited by Jesse M. Pines, Jameel Abualenain, James Scott and Robert Shesser.
© 2014 John Wiley & Sons, Ltd. Published 2014 by John Wiley & Sons, Ltd.

- *Errors in prevention* through inadequate preventive care or follow-up of treatment; or
- *Errors in systems* that provide the infrastructure for care delivery.

These domains are also implicated in emergency medicine. The primary source of error in emergency medicine closed malpractice claims is failure of diagnosis, followed by improper performance of a procedure, and delay in patient care.[2] Process-related delays in medication delivery and diagnostic testing have been identified as the most common culprits of non-ideal care events in the ED.[3] Furthermore, inexperienced ED providers are more likely to make medical errors.[4]

In order to further understand and thereby decrease medical errors, the Joint Commission mandates that hospitals identify sentinel events (serious medical errors or near misses) and determine the root causes so that quality improvements in health care delivery can be made. Three root cause categories have consistently been identified as major contributors to medical error:[5]

1 *Human factors* errors include inadequate or inadequately skilled staff, lack of staff orientation to the workplace and equipment, inadequate supervision of staff and junior physicians, inadequate competency assessment or inappropriate credentialing, and workload issues such as fatigue and distraction.

2 *Leadership* errors include poor organizational planning, resource allocation, and service integration, a lack of or lack of adherence to policies and clinical practice guidelines, and a culture tolerant of error.

3 *Communication* errors include inaccurate, incomplete, or lack of oral, written, or electronic communications amongst members of the health care team and the patient or family.

In summary, inadequate individual skills, failures in team work and communications, or gaps in infrastructure and environmental support can lead to flawed performance and poor patient outcomes. These problems are exacerbated when the medical event in question is rare, or taxes the capabilities of the health care system – as is frequently the case in EDs. Medical education must address the technical, communications, and leadership skills required to improve the health care environment and ensure better patient outcomes in critical care areas.

## Learning concepts related to improving patient outcomes

Rapid advances in medical knowledge, technology, and treatment options require medical practitioners to revise their practice considerations frequently. For example, data regarding the relative efficacy of chest compressions and ventilation in cardiac arrest patients have changed the priorities and delivery of resuscitative care over the last 5 years. Thus, medical education must teach not only content, but also the acquisition of new knowledge in a self-directed goal-oriented manner. Knowles developed the concept of andragogy to describe learning in adults who are self-directed, build on life experiences to support their learning, have learning needs related to changing social roles, are learning for the purpose of immediate application, and are motivated to learn by internal pressures (self-improvement) rather than external expectations.[6]

Active learning requires an individual to participate in the learning process by applying or extending existing knowledge to a new problem or situation, engaging the problem, and observing and reflecting on the results.[7] Active learning is based in constructivist theory which suggests that an individual must test the environment – for example, care for a critically ill patient or perform a life-saving procedure – to develop adequate knowledge of the domain. Active learning is an ideal vehicle to help medical practitioners translate theoretical knowledge into practical bedside skills, particularly in the action-oriented emergency medicine domain.

Deliberate practice is the concept that practice is most effective when trainees attempt to improve performance of a given task with every repetition.[8] The task is divided into discrete steps, each with pre-defined expert performance standards. Performance feedback is immediate, and can be provided by an external expert, or obtained more actively through debriefing in which learners reflect on their own performance in a facilitated goal-oriented discussion.

A closely associated concept, mastery learning, proposes that learners must achieve competence in all aspects of a task before training is complete. Progress towards mastery is learner-dependent, and may require a variety of educational modalities and variable time commitments for individuals to achieve success. The endpoint of training becomes total skill mastery, rather than a predefined training time or a range of passing scores.[9]

## Evaluation of educational efficacy in health care

In order to be sustainable, innovations in medical education must demonstrate value to the health care field. The gold standard, improved patient health, can be difficult to demonstrate and even more difficult to link to an isolated educational intervention. The concept of translational research, the process of moving bench research to the clinical realm, has been applied to simulation education to provide a framework for assessing its clinical impact. Laboratory research (T1) requires objective demonstration that a learner's knowledge or skills has improved. Efficacy research (T2) evaluates the impact of training on health care delivery through surrogate markers such as number of procedural attempts or time required to perform a diagnostic test. Outcomes research (T3) demonstrates improved health outcomes for individuals or groups of patients.[10]

## History of medical simulation

The first medical simulator widely used for education was "La Machine," a fabric, wicker, and leather birthing simulator developed by Madame du Coudray in eighteenth century France, which the inventor used to train midwives throughout the country at the request of Louis XV. Modern medical simulation originated in the 1960s with the development of the iconic Resusci Annie rescue-breathing simulator.[11] Medical simulation's growth in the twentieth century was largely supported by the military, which had noted dramatic cost and life savings from the implementation of Edward Link's cockpit trainer and sought to transfer the lessons learned in aviation to medicine.

Resusci Annie was the first modern partial task trainer, and its descendants are still widely used in the training of cardiopulmonary resuscitation (CPR). Partial task trainers enable clinicians to practice selected steps of a procedure in isolation, with the goal of improving psychomotor skills. Commercially available static models – anatomic representations produced from synthetic materials – exist for many common and critical bedside procedures, including vascular access, CPR, lumbar puncture, thoracentesis and paracentesis, airway management, and wound care. Educational curricula and skills evaluations are provided by the instructor. More advanced computerized task trainers provide wraparound educational content, track performance metrics, and provide automated feedback to learners – thus providing consistent instruction to all learners and reducing demands on faculty time.

The first computerized full-scale human body simulator, Sim 1, was developed in the 1960s with support of the aviation industry, and used initially for anesthesia training.[11] The cost of the single handmade simulator was prohibitive, and widespread use of full body simulators occurred only after the advent of more cost-effective models in the late 1980s. Current models incorporate variable cardiopulmonary findings (pulses, breathing, heart and lung sounds) and support performance of select emergency procedures such as airway management, defibrillation, and vascular access. Specialty-specific models for trauma, obstetric, and pediatric care also exist. These mannequins are used to simulate patients in time-sensitive scenarios so that individuals and teams of health care providers can practice care delivery in an urgent environment.

Software-based simulation programs require and respond to user input, teaching fundamental knowledge, sequencing of tasks, and prioritization. Examples include the American Heart Association's HeartCode ACLS program which enables users to practice the individual cognitive skills of a resuscitation team leader. The University of Florida's anesthesia portfolio (UFL) provides animated lung and ventilator loops to illustrate gas delivery, effects of medication, and machine controls.[12] Virtual worlds such as Second Life (www.secondlife.com), an online interactive environment, enable a user's avatar (virtual representation) to interact with other avatars and structures in the virtual environment. Larger immersive simulation rooms project images and sound around the learner to create a life-size virtual world.

Standardized patients, individuals taught to act as a patient, were first conceptualized in 1963 by neurologist Howard Barrows.[13] Dr Barrows trained a clinical assistant to demonstrate pertinent neurologic findings so that he could assess medical student performance in a reproducible fashion. Standardized patients are now routinely used in medical education to train communications and examination skills, and are used to evaluate medical students as a component of required medical licensure examinations in the United States.

## Improving care through simulation

Simulation allows learners to engage fully in active learning without fear of harming a patient. This safe environment fosters exploration, and encourages reflection, repetition, and deliberate practice. Simulation training has been demonstrated to improve the knowledge, skills, quality of care delivery, and efficiency of health care providers, as well as demonstrate positive effects on patient-related outcomes, over a broad range of training applications.[14]

## Procedural skills training

Bedside procedural skills such as insertion of a central venous catheter (CVC) have traditionally been learned through the "see one, do one, teach one model" in which a novice practitioner first observes, then performs, and finally teaches the procedure to another practitioner. Poor outcomes, financial pressure from insurance providers, and educated consumer demands for highly skilled practitioners have limited this practice.

Simulation-based procedural skills curricula have been implemented and demonstrated to have value at the T1, T2, and T3 levels. Trainees who completed a deliberate practice-based curriculum for placement of CVCs demonstrated superior skills performance on a 27-item checklist when compared with traditionally trained colleagues (T1).[15] Similar laboratory-based studies have demonstrated the efficacy of deliberate practice and mastery learning on the performance of other common ED procedures including lumbar puncture, paracentesis, thoracentesis, conscious sedation, and ACLS algorithm adherence.[16–21] Clinicians trained to mastery standards for CVC insertion required fewer needle passes to perform the procedure than traditionally trained peers (T2), and reported fewer adverse events and higher procedure success rates (T3), thus demonstrating both improved delivery of care and better patient outcomes.[22-24] Cost savings associated with reductions in CVC-related bloodstream infections are estimated to be substantial.[25]

However, the evaluation of most simulation-based procedural skills training is not rigorous. Trainee satisfaction or self-reported improvement in knowledge and confidence are often used as surrogate markers for efficacy. Without validation that a skills training program improves objective skills performance, care delivery, or patient outcomes, the value of the educational sessions is difficult to assess. Standard metrics of success with which to determine procedural training efficacy using simulation are required.

## Teamwork training

A teamwork failure occurs when skilled practitioners with adequate clinical resources fail to deliver high-quality care. The concept of Crisis Resource Management (CRM) in health care was adapted from the aviation industry's Crew Resource Management, a training program for flight crews developed to counteract the high proportion of teamwork failures implicated in airline crashes.[26] CRM principles have been modified for the health care environment, most notably by the Agency for Healthcare Research and Quality in the form of TeamSTEPPS, a freely available team training program that promotes high-quality team behavior and communication skills. The key principles of CRM and TeamSTEPPS require that team members:[27]

• Maintain *situational awareness* of the patient's status, the progress of the care team, and any unexpected obstacles to care delivery.
• Create a *shared mental model* so that all team members understand the patient's current status and plan of care.
• Provide *effective leadership* by making appropriate care and task assignment decisions, and incorporating team member input when appropriate.
• *Communicate effectively* using concise but explicit language to convey situational cues and suggestions for clinical action.
• *Allocate resources* (including staff) appropriately.
• *Provide mutual support* to team members who need assistance.

The integration of full body mannequins into team behavior training curricula creates a unique active learning environment. Simulation sessions are based on real medical scenarios and are conducted in realistic health care environments. Sessions are recorded and the video is used to support post-scenario debriefing, which reviews objective performance criteria such as delays in medication administration or failed procedures as well as teamwork skills review. Individuals deliberately practice team behaviors in successive simulation cases with the goal of providing efficient and timely clinical care.

Clinically efficient teams are more likely to use content-rich closed loop communications, employ a coordinated approach to task completion, and allocate tasks appropriately.[28] Team behaviors (T1) improved after simulation-based team training (SBTT) in interdisciplinary trauma care,[29,30] adult and neonatal resuscitation,[31,32] and obstetric emergency training.[33] Care delivery, measured using surrogate markers such as the time to complete the primary survey, intubation, defibrillation, transport to CT scanner, or degree of adherence to clinical care guidelines (ACLS) also improved with SBTT in both simulation (T1)[29–31] and clinical care (T2) environments.[29,30]

Few studies demonstrate improved patient outcomes (T3) with SBTT. After team training exercises using sentinel event cases from a pediatric ED were implemented, the frequency of adverse patient safety events decreased threefold, from 12 events in 5 years to two events in 7 years (T3).[16] Mortality rates of deteriorating pediatric patients in a tertiary children's hospital declined after instantiation of a medical emergency team which supported weekly SBTT and included leaners from all wards of the hospital.[17] Pediatric survival rates after in-hospital cardiopulmonary arrest in a tertiary care academic medical center improved from 33% to 56% with the implementation of simulated pediatric resuscitation "mock codes" that incorporated both procedural and team skills debriefing.[18] Neonatal injury rates have also been reduced using both procedural and team skills training.[19,33]

## Environmental assessment

Simulation can be used to identify physical plant deficiencies in the clinical arena. Environmental barriers to high-quality health care can be attributed to medication, equipment, or system/resource issues. Medication errors can result from poor labeling, proximate storage of look-alike medications, or complex medication administration requirements. Examples of equipment-related delays include variations in resuscitation room layout, defibrillator models, and code cart contents between different rooms in the same health care facility. Resource issues include lack of adequate staffing or availability of clinical decision tools at the bedside. *In situ* simulation training can be used to identify and correct these environmental threats before real patients are harmed.[20,21]

## Disaster preparedness

Major incidents are defined as events whose impact exceeds routine capacity. A large influx of high acuity patients into an ED taxes providers, infrastructure, and ancillary services; delays in care can worsen patient outcomes. Simulated events that test ED response are variable in design.

Table-top exercises are inexpensive but do not capture systems failures related to physical implementation of emergency plans. Mass casualty simulations using standardized patient and full body simulators enable hospitals to evaluate existing procedures and resources for resiliency, but are expensive and resource intensive.[22] In addition, disruption of routine clinical services for simulation events puts current patients at risk. Low-cost computer-based virtual worlds such as Second Life can be used to create the various environments associated with a major incident, and have been well received as they are sufficiently realistic to support both the procedural and team skills training and assessment domains.[23–25] There are no data to suggest optimal scope or frequency of disaster training.

## Conclusions

Simulation is a powerful tool for education and quality improvement in emergency medicine, and simulation-based curricula have demonstrated improved health care outcomes in select domains. However, significant translational research gaps still exist. Validated mastery standard performance has not been identified for many critical procedural skills, and team training effects research is in its infancy. In addition, the use of simulation to refine individual providers' cognitive skills, judgment, and decision-making in critical care environments using active learning and deliberate practice constructs should be explored.[34]

Demonstration of procedural skills mastery will become integral to credentialing (receiving approval to perform a skill or task in the clinical setting) in the near future. Many health care facilities already require mastery standard performance of airway management and CVC insertion skills for trainees or newly certified physicians. As simulation technology and performance metrics mature, simulation credentialing requirements are likely to expand. In addition, simulation training may become part of the national certification processes for emergency medicine practitioners. In fact, simulation training has already been incorporated in the American Society of Anesthesia's maintenance of certification program as a required component of continuing medical education.

Skills maintenance is not automatic. The optimal training frequency required to maintain team and procedural skills competence has not been established, and will clearly vary by task and trainee. Decisions regarding training frequency should be evidence-based as they will impact re-credentialing and certification processes and requirements.

Newer simulation models will enhance the simulation experience. Advances in materials technology will improve simulator realism, and highly developed curricular content and validated evaluation tools will improve the efficiency of simulation training. As health care spending becomes more proscribed, the need to demonstrate quantifiably the efficacy of a training program will drive the direction of simulation in emergency care.

## References

1 Kohn LT; the Institute of Medicine Committee on the Quality of Healthcare in America. To err is human: building a safer health system. National Academy of Sciences. 1999.

2 Brown TW, McCarthy ML, Kelen GD, Levy F. An epidemiologic study of closed emergency department malpractice claims in a national database of physician malpractice insurers. Acad Emerg Med. 2010;17:553–60.

3 Hall KK, Schenkel SM, Hirshon JM, Xiao Y, Noskin GA. Incidence and types of non-ideal care events in an emergency department. Qual Saf Health Care. 2010;19(Suppl 3):i20–5.

4 Berk WA, Welch RD, Levy PD, Jones JT, Arthur C, Kuhn GJ, et al. The effect of clinical experience on the error rate of emergency physicians. Ann Emerg Med. 2008;52(5):497–501.

5 Joint Commission. Root causes of sentinel events by event type. Available at: http://www.jointcommission.org/assets/1/18/Root_Causes_Event_Type_04_4Q2012.pdf (accessed 29 November 2013).

6 Merriam SB (ed.) The New Update on Adult Learning Theory: New Directions for Adult and Continuing Education. New York: Jossey-Bass, John Wiley and Sons Inc, 2001.

7 Graffam B. Active learning in medical education: strategies for beginning implementation. Med Teach. 2007;29:38–42.

8 Ericsson KA. Deliberate practice and acquisition of expert performance: a general overview. Acad Emerg Med. 2008;15:988–94.

9 McGaghie WC, Issenberg SB, Cohen ER, Barsuk JH, Wayne DB. Medical education featuring mastery learning with deliberate practice can lead to better health for individuals and populations. Acad Med. 2011;86(11):e8–9.

10 McGaghie WC. Medical education research as translational science. Sci Transl Med. 2010;2(19):19cm8.

11 Rosen KR. The history of medical simulation. J Crit Care 2008;23:157–66.

12 University of Florida's Simulation Portfolio. Available at: http://vam.anest.ufl.edu/simulations/simulationportfolio.php (accessed 29 November 2013).

13 Wallace P. Following the threads of an innovation: the history of standardized patients in medical education. Caduceus. 1997;13(2):5–28.

14 Cook DA, Hatala R, Brydges R, Zendejas B, Szostek JH, Wang AT, et al. Technology-enhanced simulation for health professions education: a systematic review and meta-analysis. J Am Med Assoc. 2011;306(9):978–88.

15 Barsuk JH, Shubhada NA, Cohen ER, McGaghie WC, Wayne DB. Mastery learning of temporary hemodialysis catheter insertion by nephrology fellows using simulation technology and deliberate practice. A J Kidney Dis. 2009;54(1):70–6.

16 Patterson MD, Geis GL, LeMaster T, Wears RL. Impact of multidisciplinary simulation-based training on patient safety in a paediatric emergency department. BMJ Qual Saf. 2013;22:383–93.

17 Theilen U, Leonard P, Jones P, Ardill R, Weitz J, Agrawal D, et al. Regular in situ simulation training of paediatric medical emergency team improves hospital response to deteriorating patients. Resuscitation. 2012;84:218–22.

18  Andreatta P, Saxton E, Thompson M, Annich G. Simulation based mock codes significantly correlate with improved pediatric patient cardiopulmonary arrest survival rates. Pediatr Crit Care Med. 2011;12:33–8.

19  Draycott TJ, Crofts JF, Ash JP. Improving neonatal outcome through practical shoulder dystocia training. Obstet Gynecol. 2008;112(1):14–20.

20  Wheeler DS, Geis G, Mack EH, LeMaster T, Patterson MD. High reliability emergency response teams in the hospital: improving quality and safety using in situ simulation training. BMJ Qual Saf. 2013;22:507–14.

21  Patterson MD, Geis GL, Falcone RA, LeMaster T, Wears RL. In situ simulation: detection of safety threats and teamwork training in a high risk emergency department. BMJ Qual Saf. 2013;22:468–77.

22  Klima DA, Seiler SH, Peterson JB, Christmas AB, Green JM, Fleming G, et al. Full-scale regional exercises: closing the gaps in disaster preparedness. J Trauma Acute Care Surg. 2012;73:592–8.

23  Andreatta PB, Maslowski E, Petty S, Shim W, Marsh M, Hall T, et al. Virtual reality triage training provides a viable solution for disaster preparedness. Acad Emerg Med. 2010;17:870–6.

24  Cohen D, Sevdalis N, Patel V, Taylor M, Lee H, Vokes M, et al. Tactical and operational response to major incidents: feasibility and reliability of skills assessment using novel virtual environments. Resuscitation. 2013;84:992–8.

25  Cohen DC, Sevdalis N, Patel V, Taylor D, Batrick N, Darzi AW. Major-incident preparation for acute hospitals: current state-of-the-art, training needs analysis, and the role of novel virtual worlds simulation technologies. J Emerg Med 2012;43(6):1029–37.

26  Carne B, Kennedy M, Gray T. Review Article: Crisis resource management in emergency medicine. Emerg Med Austral. 2012;24:7–13.

27  Agency for Healthcare Research and Quality. TeamSTEPPS. Available at: http://teamstepps.ahrq.gov/ (accessed 29 November 2013).

28  Siassakos D, Bristowe K, Draycott TJ, Angouri J, Hambly H, Winter C, et al. Clinical efficiency in a simulated emergency and relationship to team behaviours: a multisite cross-sectional study. BJOG 2001;118:596–607.

29  Steinemann S, Berg B, Skinner A, DiTulio A, Anzelon K, Terada K, et al. In situ, multidisciplinary, simulation-based teamwork training improves early trauma care. J Surg Ed. 2011;68:472–7.

30  Capella J, Smith S, Philp A, Putnam T, Gilbert C, Fry W, et al. Teamwork training improves the clinical care of trauma patients. J Surg. 2010;67:439–43.

31  Davita MA, Schaefer J, Lutz J, Wang H, Dongilli T. Improving medical emergency team (MET) performance using a novel curriculum and a computerized human patient simulator. Qual Saf Health Care. 2005;14:326–31.

32  Sawyer T, Laubach VA, Hudak J, Yamamura K, Pocrnich A. Improvements in teamwork during neonatal resuscitation after interprofessional teamSTEPPS training. Neonatal Netw. 2013;32(1):26–33.

33  Grobman WA, Miller D, Burke C, Hornbogen A, Tam K, Costello R. Outcomes associated with introduction of a shoulder dystocia protocol. Am J Obstetr Gynecol. 2011;205(6):513–7.

34  McGaghie WC, Draycott TJ, Dunn WF, Lopez CM, Stefanidis D. Evaluating the impact of simulation on translational patient outcomes. Simul Healthc. 2011;6(Suppl):S42–7.

# PART 3

# Emergency care workforce

# CHAPTER 8

# Emergency care workforce projections

## James Scott[1], Rachelle Pierre-Mathew[2], and Drew Maurano[2]

[1]Department of Emergency Medicine and Health Policy, The George Washington University, USA
[2]Department of Emergency Medicine, The George Washington University, USA

## Rapid growth of ED utilization

The explosion of demand for emergency services by the US population is often ascribed to a failure of the health care system to provide adequate preventive and primary care. However, an alternative explanation is that the evolution of the modern emergency department (ED) is a great success story as the dramatic increase in ED utilization reflects the recognition of the quality and value of ED services by patients and providers.

In the early 1960s, when designated EDs were first being described, virtually all hospitals had an "emergency room." These were small, often inaccessible areas of the hospital which operated haphazardly in a nonstandardized fashion. If EDs were open after hours or on weekends they were operating within a hospital that was otherwise closed. Access to radiology, laboratory services, and timely consultation were unavailable in virtually any of these units. The physicians and nurses who staffed these emergency rooms were not formally trained in emergency care and often reluctantly provided these services in exchange for continued hospital privileges or a supplement to their base pay.

Fast forward to 2013 and virtually every hospital has a fully functioning ED that provides a full scope of services 24 hours a day, 7 days a week, 365 days a year. Sophisticated imaging, laboratory studies, and stabilization and resuscitation are available within minutes. More complex magnetic resonance imaging, interventional radiology, or surgical procedures can almost always be arranged within a few hours.

*Emergency Care and The Public's Health*, First Edition.
Edited by Jesse M. Pines, Jameel Abualenain, James Scott and Robert Shesser.
© 2014 John Wiley & Sons, Ltd. Published 2014 by John Wiley & Sons, Ltd.

Many reasons have been proposed for the increase in the utilization of emergency services, but perhaps the most important is that the modern ED provides high-quality, reliable care in a very timely manner. EDs bring all of the available resources of a technologically equipped hospital to the patient at the time that the patient and the ED physician determine that it is needed. It is fair to say that there is no other place with the depth and breadth of capabilities anywhere else in the health care system. The fact that patients demand and now expect this care is not surprising.

If we only examine the "modern" era, there has been an almost 50% increase in ED visits. In 1990 there were approximately 90 million ED visits in the United States and it is predicted that by 2015 there will be more than 140 million visits. To put this in perspective, the US population has increased by approximately 20% during that period. Since the 1970s there has been almost a 400% increase in ED visits while the US population has increased by approximately 10% per decade.[1]

Increased ED visits have occurred despite purposeful, systematic, directed attempts to decrease ED usage. With the advent of managed care, it was assumed that with more coordinated and active primary care for their patients, the utilization of emergency services for primary care sensitive conditions would decrease. Managed care assigned gatekeepers whose prospective approval for emergency services use was needed. It now remains to be seen if the current emphasis on patient-centered medical homes or accountable care organizations will slow the growth of emergency care utilization.

Part of the ED utilization growth was encouraged by the Emergency Treatment and Active Labor Act (EMTALA) which was enacted in the mid-1980s and required that hospitals provide unfettered access to emergency care for all individuals regardless of their insurance status or ability to pay. This mandate to provide care for all comers is unique to hospital EDs and not required anywhere else in the US healthcare system. While this legislation has had some small effect on the behavior of hospitals, and minimal effect on emergency physicians, the US population now understands that access to emergency care is one of their legal rights.

Virtually all large hospital EDs report double-digit increases during the last 10 years due both to aforementioned increase in ED visits nationally and the 10% decease in the number of hospitals with active EDs[2] This has served to concentrate the volume of patients into a smaller number of departments which have grown in size, but are now often stretched to the limits of their resources and staffing.

We live in a society that has become unaccustomed to waiting. EDs are good providers of high technology-oriented care, albeit financially inefficient in their current configuration. When high-quality resource-intense care is available 24 hours a day without appointment, and every person in the country knows this and also knows it is their legal right to access that care regardless their ability to pay, it is not only understandable but completely predictable that the ED utilization would increase.

## Population growth and changing demographics

The US population is expected to increase dramatically over the next several decades. Current estimates predict that it will reach nearly 438 million people in 2050.[3] This number is a marked increase from the US reported census of 310 million Americans in 2010.[4] Providing high-quality and accessible health care for this growing population poses a challenge to our society. As the population continues to increase, EDs may continue to experience a growing patient census.[5]

The expected population explosion over the next several decades includes increases in the elderly and immigrant populations.[4] The aging of the "baby boomer" cohort, accounts for the projected increase in the elderly population. In 2030, almost 20% of the US population will be above the age of 65. This will include an increase from 35 million seniors in 2000 to a projected 72 million in 2030. This longevity will result in an increased prevalence of chronic diseases and will strain the nation's healthcare resources and threaten the financial viability of entitlement programs like Medicare. The growing older adult population will increase the number of elderly patients seen in EDs.[6] Over the past two decades, EDs nationwide have already seen a rise in the number of visits by older adult patients.[7] Older adult patients in the ED are more likely than younger patients to have longer lengths of stay, use more resources, and require admission.[8] In addition, geriatric patients have a higher morbidity and mortality.[9] As ED providers continue to provide a larger share of geriatric services, special consideration will need to be targeted towards the complex social and medical needs of elderly patients.

The US population increase will also be a result of an influx of immigrants and their descendants.[3] Nearly 20% of all Americans in 2050 will be recent immigrants, compared to 12% in 2005. This increase will also include a marked shift to a larger Latino population. As the population continues to diversify, emergency health care providers will be challenged to provide not only more quality care, but culturally competent and appropriate care. Overall, this diverse and aging population explosion will bestow unique challenges to an already complex and overtaxed emergency health care system.

As healthcare utilization increases, the ED may experience early manifestations of systemic overload through increased crowding.[10] ED patients treated in a crowded environment have more frequent treatment delays and greater morbidity and mortality than patients in less crowded

ED conditions.[11,12] Treatment delays lead to increased length of stay for both admitted and discharged patients.[13] ED crowding is also associated with an increase in medical errors.[14] Hospitals with crowded EDs are often forced to divert ambulances to other hospitals, which can delay patient treatment and hamper the ability to transport new patients.[12] Furthermore, crowding has a negative impact on patient satisfaction, can erode patient confidentiality, and contributes to burnout and increased staff turnover.

## Effect of ACA on ED utilization

In an attempt to improve health care quality, expand access, and control costs, the Affordable Care Act (ACA) was enacted in 2010.[15] The ACA will expand health insurance access to over 32 million Americans.[16] This expansion will be a combination of private insurance obtained through health insurance exchanges and the expansion of Medicaid.[15] Amidst projections of population growth, a growing elderly population, and the ACA insurance expansion, the United States is expected to need nearly 52 000 new primary care physicians by 2025. Although it is unknown how many new emergency physicians will be needed,[17] there is growing concern that more patients will turn to EDs to access health care. Furthermore, concerns have been raised that the approximately 16 million new Medicaid beneficiaries will also be high users of ED care.[18] Traditionally, Medicaid patients utilize EDs at twice the rate of uninsured and privately insured patients.[19] One proposed reason is that the traditionally low Medicaid reimbursement rates have created a barrier for beneficiaries to access primary care. The ACA attempts to counteract this barrier by increasing primary care provider reimbursement rates to the level of Medicare reimbursement.[15] It remains to be seen what effect, if any, the primary care workforce expansion and Medicaid reimbursement increase within the ACA will have on primary care access and ED utilization.

Recent healthcare reform efforts in Massachusetts have been studied as a potential model for ACA-induced system requirements nationwide. In 2006, Massachusetts enacted health reform measures to decrease the number of uninsured patients.[20] These reform efforts later served as a template for drafting the ACA.[21] The Massachusetts experience is inconclusive as to whether the ACA will lead to an increase or decrease ED utilization.[22] After coverage expansion, ED visits in Massachusetts increased, but this increase was at the same rate as that experienced in neighboring states which did not expand insurance coverage.[23] There has been speculation that the cause of the increase has been inadequate primary care access, less cost-sharing for emergency services, or population growth.[22] However, it is difficult to attribute this increase to one specific cause and it is likely multifactorial and mirrors national trends. Although frequent users of the ED are not a homogenous group, research has shown that the majority of high users of ED care are often sick patients with chronic illnesses and high rates of admission.[24] As previously noted, the common misconception that ambulatory sensitive primary care visits are the leading drivers of ED utilization is false and efforts to decrease these visit have had little impact on ED crowding.[21]

## Current and predicted ED workforce numbers

In 2009 there were approximately 39 000 emergency physicians practicing in EDs in the United States.[25] With approximately 1500 emergency medicine residents graduating each year and predicted retirement of 3% of emergency physicians per year, the workforce will add 330 net emergency physicians for a growth rate of 0.8% per year. When compared with the historical growth of the demand for emergency medicine services (EMS) this leaves a potential shortfall of thousands of practicing emergency physicians. If the actual retirement rate for today's older emergency physicians is greater than 3%, the shortfall will be even greater.

While there are no clear data on emergency medicine nursing supply, according the National Bureau of Labor Statistics, there were an estimated 2.7 million registered nurses within the United States in 2010.[26] This number is expected to increase by 26% in 2020 to approximately 3.4 million registered nurses. Despite the continued increase in the number of RNs, there have been various predictions of whether the nursing supply can meet future demand for care. The Health Resources and Services Administration (HRSA) predicts a full-time equivalent (FTE) shortfall as high as 1 million nurses in 2020.[27,28] The predicted shortages are multifactorial; however, a rapidly aging workforce that will soon be facing retirement has been cited as a major contributor to the shortage, especially in a field as demanding as emergency medicine. As the first generation of emergency physicians ages it is more common to see veteran physicians in the ED, but the presence of seasoned nurses, especially on difficult night and weekend shifts, is increasingly rare.

The Bureau of Labor Statistics predicts that physician assistants (PAs) will be the second-fastest-growing profession in the next decade, increasing from 74 800 in 2008 to 103 900 in 2018. The American Academy of Physician Assistants (AAPA) projects that in 2020 there will be 137 000–173 000 certified PAs.[29] If the current percentage of PAs practicing emergency medicine remains at 11%, there could be as many as 10 000 new PAs practicing emergency medicine a decade from now.[30] While this will certainly provide some buffer to the expected physician shortfall, it will certainly require some modifications in practice and management.

## Current models of emergency department staffing

The current emergency health system includes pre-hospital components, urban and rural community hospitals, academic medical centers, specialty EDs such as pediatric and psychiatric EDs, and local and regional trauma centers. Widely fluctuating daily and hourly patient volume, acuity, and demographics further complicate the process of "right sizing" ED staffing. Optimal and safe ED staffing algorithms are complex and solutions designed for other service industries or other sectors of healthcare often fail in the ED.

The FTEs needed to staff an ED is comprised of both nursing and physician elements. Calculating the number of staff depends on many factors: space, volume, peaks in volume, acuity, patient safety, cost, and department protocols. Significant research is focused on identifying the barriers that affect the ED system's ability to provide care and move patients through the system. Numerous models and strategic drivers have been created to guide the staffing of the ED. Most EDs require a charge nurse, triage nurse, one nurse per 3–5 active patients, and ancillary resources such as radiology and laboratory technicians.[31] This standard model is then expanded based on length of stay, boarding patients, acuity, and specialty services available. Conversely, the physician model is based the number of patients an individual can evaluate and treat an hour. The average board-certified emergency physician can see 2.3–2.8 patients per hour.[32] Therefore most groups calculate physician staffing by arrival volumes, which may not account for acuity, length of stay, wait times, boarding rates, procedural time, and provider variation. The volume on a given day can fluctuate up to 40% by time of arrival, with most of the patients arriving at the ED between 10 a.m. and 10 p.m. The introduction of electronic health records (EHRs) may adversely impact some EDs by reducing physician productivity to 1.8–2.8 patients per hour.[33]

ED staffing must balance the need to flexibly respond to volume changes while minimizing operational costs. If an ED overstaffs, the net income per patient encounter will decrease. Many administrators staff based on 24-hour average volumes despite great variability in the hourly arrival patterns. During some hours, 10 patients may present, and at other hours only 1–2 patients present. Staffing with ED technicians and other lower cost, non-registered nurse (RN) positions allows nurses to focus on uniquely nursing functions, providing assistance for high volume periods at lower cost, as it is estimated that 14% of ED nursing tasks can be accomplished by non-RN personnel.[34]

PAs and nurse practitioners (NPs) have recently been integrated into the ED as a way to decrease the number of physicians needed. PAs practice medicine with the supervision of a licensed physician, and although by law PAs are dependent practitioners, they typically exercise considerable autonomy in clinical decision-making. Supervision is defined by each state, and may be provided by varied methods such as physical presence or reasonable access by telephone or electronic media.

NPs are advanced practicing nurses who are trained to provide a range of advanced health services for a particular subset of the population. NPs can be trained in family medicine, adult medicine, pediatric, neonatal, geriatric, obstetrics and gynecology, oncology, mental health, and acute care. The family medicine and adult medicine NPs have been utilized in the urgent care and fast track ED models. The acute care NP has been used in the higher acuity sections of EDs with success. The limiting factor is the narrow training of each subset which prohibits practice, such as an adult medicine NP working in an ED cannot treat a pediatric patient. The role of the NP nationally continues to change as the education requirement moves towards the Doctor of Nursing Practice (DNP). The number of subsets of training continues to grow as has the autonomy granted to these advanced practice nurses. There has been a national discussion concerning the advisability of combining the family medicine and acute care tracks to produce a specific emergency trained NP.

PA training follows the physician model and is broad enough to manage the complete spectrum of cases that present to the ED. NPs are independent providers and in some cases are less dependent on the ED attending physician. Most hospital systems credential both providers in the same way and require some level of physician supervision for both. Medicare and some private insurance companies reimburse care billed by PAs and NPs at 85% of the physician rate. Visits that are managed jointly in real time by the physician and PA or NP are reimbursed at 100% of the physician rate.

PAs, NPs, or both are being used 68.5% of the time in main EDs as primary providers, 19.4% in fast tracks, 11.4% in urgent cases, and 0.73% for initial triage.[35] The best cost–benefit is the use of the PA or NP on the fast track solely without a physician. Fast track patients typically present with primary or urgent care-based complaints often resulting in lower E and M coding levels. These codes are reimbursed at a work relative value unit (RVU) of 0.6–1.77. Depending on the conversion factor used, these providers will average $28.9 per RVU compared to physicians at $33.97 per RVU.[36] In comparing revenue to median salaries, a board certified emergency medicine physician earns approximately $250 000 compared to $103 000 for that of an ED trained PA or NP. Efficient use of these providers also allows physicians to delegate procedures and time-consuming tasks which then enables the physician to focus on evaluating more patients, managing complex patient care, and documentation.

ED scribes are adjunct personnel who assist in tasks for which physicians have been traditionally responsible, especially charting in eletronic health records. A scribe helps the physician to increase patient contact time, give more thought to complex cases, better manage patient flow through the department, and increase productivity to see more patients. Physicians working without a scribe average 2.3–2.8 patients per hour compared to 3.1 per hour with scribes.[37] At an average increase of 1.5 RVUs an hour, the use of a scribe results in a net gain of $40–55 per hour. A trained scribe makes $9–$25 per hour and not only increases reimbursement, but decreases ED length of stay, increases compliance with core measure documentation, and increases physician satisfaction.

Alternative ED staffing models are just one approach to better matching supply and demand of resources.

In the last decade, healthcare systems have attempted to provide alternatives for ED patients by opening freestanding EDs with all the traditional resources of a hospital-based ED but without the inpatient capability or specialty consultation available on site. The freestanding emergency center has the potential to improve access to care as it may be located closer to the patient's home or place of work. Data are lacking to determine the impact on reducing overall emergency visits or overall manpower needs.

CVS Caremark Corporation, the largest pharmacy healthcare provider in the United States launched the first retail medical clinic in 2000 and currently has approximately 600 locations in 25 states and the District of Columbia. Nationally, the company has cared for more than 13 million patients with a 95% customer satisfaction rating.[38] The CVS MinuteClinic focuses on the urgent care patient who is unable to see their physician, has limited access to a physician, and requires minimal testing. These clinics are staffed by advanced practice nurses. No data are yet available on comparative productivity of an advanced practice nurse in an ED versus that in a retail setting, so the impact of these clinics on overall healthcare manpower needs is unclear.

## Potential future models

In the near future it may be necessary to acknowledge that not all EDs need to be the same or deliver the same level of care. Similar to the freestanding ED or the designated trauma pyramid (Levels I–III), it may be time to create a graded system of emergency care. In some jurisdictions this is already in place for trauma and cardiac care. It could be argued that the growth of retail-based walk-in clinics and freestanding EDs has created this by default. If this system were coordinated so patients and EMS providers knew what services were available where, and provided by whom, it could provide a system for much better matching of the patent's medical needs and the resources and expertise of the provider and facility, thus reducing the overall emergency services manpower requirements.

Alternatively, if primary, urgent, and emergency services were co-located, patients could be immediately directed to the appropriate level of care. NPs administering immunizations or refilling medications and general urgent care, primary care physicians providing longitudinal care and management alterations, and emergency physicians and PAs providing true emergency care in the same facility. The matching of the patients' needs to the capabilities of the individual providers should decrease the manpower needs and lead to greater efficiency.

The utilization of emergency services has increased dramatically and there is little reason to expect that the demand will abate any time soon. Many attempts to limit or discourage the use of EDs by more and more patients have failed, and there is strong evidence to suggest that, by virtue of demographics, disease patterns, and access, the need for emergency care will only continue to increase. The answer may be more emergency physicians, nurses, mid-level providers, technicians, and scribes, but new organizational structures are needed to optimize system efficiency.

## References

1 United States Department of Health and Human Services. Centers for Disease Control and Prevention. National Center for Health Statistics. National Hospital Ambulatory Medical Care Survey, 2008. ICPSR29922-v1. Ann Arbor, MI: Inter-university Consortium for Political and Social Research. 2011.

2 Ginde A, Sullivan A, Camargo C. National Study of Emergency Physician Workforce. Ann Emerg Med. 2009; 54:349–59.

3 Passel JS, Chon DV. US Population Projections: 2005–2050. Pew Research Center, 2008.

4 Vincent GK,Velkoff VA. The Next Four Decades, The Older Population in the United States: 2010 to 2050, Current Population Reports. US Census Bureau, 2010.

5 Tang N, Stein J, Hsia RY, Maselli JH, Gonzales R. Trends and characteristics of US emergency department visits, 1997–2007. J Am Med Assoc 2010; 304(6):664–70.

6 Xu KT, Nelson BK, Berk S. The changing profile of patients who used emergency department services in the United States: 1996 to 2005. Ann Emerg Med. 2009; 54(6):805–10, e1–7.

7 Roberts DC, McKay MP, Shaffer A. Increasing rates of emergency department visits for elderly patients in the United States, 1993 to 2003. Ann Emerg Med. 2008; 51(6):769–74.

8 Strange GR, Chen EH, Sanders AB. Use of emergency departments by elderly patients: projections from a multicenter data base. Ann Emerg Med. 1992; 21(7):819–24.

9 Aminzadeh F, Dalziel WB. Older adults in the emergency department: a systematic review of patterns of use, adverse outcomes, and effectiveness of interventions. Ann Emerg Med. 2002; 39(3):238–47.

10 Institute of Medicine. Hospital-Based Emergency Care: At the Breaking Point. National Academies Press, 2006.

11 Bernstein SL, Aronsky D, Duseja R, Epstein S, Handel D, Hwang U, et al. The effect of emergency department crowding on clinically oriented outcomes. Acad Emerg Med. 2009; 16(1):1–10.

12 Boyle A, Beniuk K, Higginson I, Atkinson P. Emergency department crowding: time for interventions and policy evaluations. Emerg Med Int. 2012; 2012:838610.

13 White BA, Biddinger PD, Chang Y, Grabowski B, Carignan S, Brown DF. Boarding inpatients in the emergency department increases discharged patient length of stay. J Emerg Med. 2012; 44:230–5.

14 Kulstad EB, Sikka R, Sweis RT, Kelley KM, Rzechula KH. ED overcrowding is associated with an increased frequency of medication errors. Am J Emerg Med. 2010; 28(3):304–9.

15 Henry J. Kaiser Family Foundation. (2011, updated 2013) Summary of new health reform law. Available at: http://kff.org/health-reform/fact-sheet /summary-of-new-health-reform-law/ (accessed 29 November 2013).

16 Marco CA, Moskop JC, Schears RM, Stankus JL, Bookman KJ, Padela AI, et al. The ethics of health care reform: impact on emergency medicine. Acad Emerg Med. 2012; 19(4):461–8.

17 Petterson SM, Liaw WR, Phillips RL Jr, Rabin DL, Meyers DS, Bazemore AW. Projecting US primary care physician workforce needs: 2010–2025. Ann Fam Med. 2012; 10(6):503–9.

18 Hotlz-Eakin D, Ramlet M. Healthcare reform and Medicaid: patient access, emergency department use, and financial implications for states and hospitals. 2010. Available at: http://www.politico.com/pdf/PPM170_hcr_medicaid.pdf (accessed 29 November 2013).

19 Peppe EM, Mays JW, Chang HC, Becker E, diJulio B. (2007) Issue brief: characteristics of frequent emergency department users. Available at: http://kaiserfamilyfoundation.files.wordpress.com/2013/01/7696.pdf (accessed 29 November 2013).

20 Long SK, Masi PB. Access and affordability: an update on health reform in Massachusetts, fall 2008. Health Aff (Millwood). 2009; 28(4):578–87.

21 Aston G. ED relief. Hosp Health Netw. 2011; 85(10):39–40, 42.

22 Chen C, Scheffler G, Chandra A. Massachusetts' health care reform and emergency department utilization. N Engl J Med. 2011; 365(12):e25.

23 Smulowitz PB, Lipton R, Wharam JF, Adelman L, Weiner SG, Burke L, et al. Emergency department utilization after the implementation of Massachusetts health reform. Ann Emerg Med. 2011; 58(3):225–234, e1.

24 LaCalle E, Rabin E. Frequent users of emergency departments: the myths, the data, and the policy implications. Ann Emerg Med. 2010; 56(1):42–8.

25  Gindi RM, Cohen RA, Kirzinger WK. Emergency Room Use Among Adults Aged 18–64: Early Release of Estimates From the National Health Interview Survey, January–June 2011. Division of Health Interview Statistics, National Center for Health Statistics, 2012.

26  Bureau of Labor Statistics, United State Department of Labor. Table 6. The 30 occupations with the largest projected employment growth, 2010–20. Available at: http://www.bls.gov/news.release/ecopro.t06.htm (accessed 29 November 2013).

27  Institute of Medicine (IOM). The Future of Nursing: Leading Change, Advancing Health. National Academies Press, 2011. Available at: http://thefutureofnursing.org/IOM-Report (accessed 29 November 2013).

28  Buerhaus PI, Auerbach DI, Staiger DO. The recent surge in nurse employment: causes and implications. Health Aff. 2009; 28(4):w657–68.

29  American Academy of Physician Assistants. Quick facts. Available at: http://www.aapa.org/the_pa_profession/quick_facts.aspx (accessed 29 November 2013).

30  American Academy of Physician Assistants. Physician Assistant Census Report. Available at: http://www.aapa.org/uploadedFiles/content/Research/2010%20Census%20Report%20National%20_Final.pdf (accessed 29 November 2013).

31  Brown R. et al. Safe nurse staffing: looking beyond the raw numbers. Vantage Point. 2009; 4:1–16.

32  Collins M. Staffing an ED appropriately and efficiently. ACEP News. 2009.

33  Schneider ME. Hospitals' unstoppable EHRs may slow their EDs. ACEP News, 2010.

34  Jagim R, Robinson KS. Nursing workforce issues and trends affecting emergency departments. Top Emerg Med. 2004; 4:276–86.

35  Society of Emergency Medicine Physician Assistants. 2009 Report of Emergency Medicine Physician Assistants. 2012.

36  Ault A. EDs search or the right midlevel provider mix. ACEP News, 2008.

37  Patel S, Rais A, Kumar A. Focus On: The Use of Scribes in the Emergency Department. American College of Emergency Physicians, 2013.

38  Our History. (2013) Available at: www.minuteclinc.com/about/history.aspx (accessed 29 November 2013).

PART 4

# Emergency preparedness and response to emergencies and disasters

CHAPTER 9

# US emergency and disaster response in the past, present, and future: The multi-faceted role of emergency health care

## Joseph A. Barbera[1] and Anthony G. Macintyre[2]

[1]*Engineering Management (Crisis and Emergency Management), Institute for Crisis, Disaster, and Risk Management, Department of Engineering Management and Systems Engineering, The George Washington University, USA*
[2]*Department of Emergency Medicine, The George Washington University, USA*

Professionals in Emergency Medicine, Emergency Nursing, Emergency Medical Services (EMS) and other emergency healthcare disciplines have played a central role in influencing how the nation responds to emergencies and disasters, and they continue to shape this challenging area. Experts from these disciplines have been at the forefront in all aspects of healthcare emergency management, including healthcare system continuity of operations, medical surge, specialty capabilities such as managing chemical casualties, and deploying medical resources into austere environments.

This chapter describes the integral roles and major influences of *Emergency Medicine* and *emergency healthcare delivery* on the past and present U.S. disaster response capabilities. These influences have occurred across all types of hazards (intentional, technological, and natural) and across all phases of comprehensive emergency management (mitigation, preparation, response, recovery). Future roles and responsibilities are also explored, including the emerging concept of Emergency Public Health as a distinct discipline, which is further described in the following chapter.

*Emergency Care and The Public's Health*, First Edition.
Edited by Jesse M. Pines, Jameel Abualenain, James Scott and Robert Shesser.
© 2014 John Wiley & Sons, Ltd. Published 2014 by John Wiley & Sons, Ltd.

## Past and present

### Health care systems

Hospitals have always had the potential to respond to emergencies and disasters. In the United States, more formalized and consistent efforts to plan for these incidents can be traced to the 1980s and early 1990s. Disaster committees were established in many hospitals by this time. In retrospect, they focused almost exclusively on relatively rudimentary preparedness, with most of the efforts centered on mass casualties arriving at the health care facility. Projections were primarily for external disaster situations and moderate numbers of blunt trauma casualties coming to their location.

Very few health care organizations conducted a formal risk assessment to develop a detailed understanding of their potential hazards and the resultant impacts that they were likely to encounter. Preparedness was generally prompted by, and oriented toward, local experience with disasters. Processes such as a formal hazards vulnerability analysis (HVA) or a business risk analysis to develop a detailed understanding of the potential hazards and their resultant impacts were not utilized.

Additionally, any attention focused on risk reduction (i.e., mitigation) was compliance-based. Few templates existed for how to organize the "disaster preparedness" body of knowledge or for how to organize the myriad related tasks. A disaster plan could vary widely in format, structure, and content from hospital to hospital, even within a jurisdiction or health care system. Many of the more formal processes have since been introduced into the health care industry by emergency health care personnel who have been schooled in formal emergency management principles. Much of this progress across the United States has been prompted by the increasingly detailed accreditation requirements of The Joint Commission (TJC), formerly the Joint Commission on Accreditation of Healthcare Organizations (JCAHO).[1]

After the worldwide attention paid to the Tokyo subway Sarin attack[2] and the Oklahoma City bombing[3] in 1995, the US government funded the Domestic Preparedness Program (DPP). A component of this consisted of widespread training for health care professionals focused on weapons of mass destruction (WMD; chemical, biological, radiological, and large-scale explosives).[4] The JCAHO also increased accreditation requirements related to mass casualties and emergencies with unusual patient injuries. Emergency health care professionals (i.e., emergency physicians, emergency nurses, emergency medical services personnel) were heavily involved with these efforts, motivated by recognition that they would be the frontline of medicine facing the dangerous and potentially overwhelming incidents associated with WMD agents.

This evolution in health care preparedness was further extended after the 2001 incidents related to the 9/11 terrorist airplane attacks and the anthrax dissemination incidents. The DPP was eclipsed by a federal program specifically focused on hospital preparedness, the National Bioterrorism Preparedness Program, which later evolved into a much more all-hazard approach as the Hospital Preparedness Program.[5] This program continues today and has funded health care organizations through State health authorities, providing metrics related to medical surge and other response requirements such as continuity of operations. An example is health care organization participation in emergency health care coalitions (EHCs) which amplify the ability for local response through mechanisms such as mutual aid between facilities.

The 2005 Hurricane Katrina impact on health care systems, in which many hospital patients and long-term care facility residents died after critical life safety systems failed,[6] refocused efforts on the importance of sustained continuity of operations in the face of a hazard impact. The resultant TJC accreditation changes required examination of an organization's ability for 96-hour self-sustainment, with much focus on inpatient services and infrastructure such as emergency electrical power. The cross-cutting understanding of patient needs by emergency personnel, however, placed them in central roles for recognizing and addressing continuity vulnerabilities.

For informed professionals working in this area, emergency preparedness has now evolved to a much more comprehensive concept of health care emergency management. It is conducted though a Comprehensive Emergency Management Program (CEMP).[7,8] CEMP recognizes all preparedness activities (Box 9.1) but also stresses risk reduction initiatives (i.e., mitigation) as well as effective guidance for response and recovery. Program activities in mitigation and preparedness are supervised by the organization's Emergency Management Committee. The concept "Emergency Management Plan," used by TJC in the late 1990s and early 2000s, which created large documents encompassing both preparedness and response guidance, has now been replaced by the common CEMP concept

---

**Box 9.1 Emergency management preparedness planning**

1 Emergency operations plan (EOP)
- Development and maintenance
- All emergency response *and* early recovery guidance
2 Preparedness resource management
- Personnel recruitment, retention, and training
- Equipment, supplies, facilities acquisition, and prep
3 Exercise and other evaluation
4 Organizational learning
- Improvement planning
- Incorporating improvements

of a streamlined and structured Emergency Operations Plan (EOP).[9] Preparedness is described separately, and the EOP incorporates incident command system structure and process to provide clear consistent response and recovery guidance. All of these activities are informed by the organization's HVA which extends beyond just hazard identification to understanding the vulnerability elements to each hazard. This is ideally described in a way that common vulnerabilities across multiple hazards can be recognized for future mitigation and preparedness action. A simple example is the commonly found vulnerability for rapid notification of staff when a hazard impact occurs or is imminent. This is encountered in a wide range of emergency situations such as tornados, patients arriving with hazardous materials contamination, and violence inside the facility. Resilient mechanisms for conveying initial notifications become important to develop and implement. Another common vulnerability involves personnel not trained to take immediate protective action in response to the danger notification, such as directed evacuation, shelter in place, or protect in place (action for an active shooter situation).

This more formal approach to health care emergency management has gradually extended beyond hospitals to other types of health care organizations. More widespread emergency management is being conducted by community health centers and other outpatient clinics, long-term care facilities, and specialty health care organizations such as dialysis centers. Many of these were prompted by publicity from Hurricane Katrina and from increasing requirements for accreditation (TJC) and reimbursement (Centers for Medicare and Medicaid Services, CMS).[10] Increasingly, the understanding of the methods and benefits may soon become the primary driver.

### Disaster medicine evolution to the broader discipline of medical and health emergency management

In parallel to evolving hospital processes and procedures, direct medical care concepts were also changing. These have been loosely described within the framework of disaster medicine. Interestingly, the evolution of disaster medicine was commonly independent of hospital planning. Many US physicians participated in the early years of the World Association for Disaster and Emergency Medicine, which was originally founded in 1976 as the Club of Mainz.[11] The first and currently largest association for emergency physicians, the American College of Emergency Physicians, also showed early formal interest with the establishment of the Disaster Medicine Section in 1989 as the first formal "section" within the College.[12] Disaster medicine focused on triage protocols, recognition of unusual disease and chemical agents, and treatment of unusual injuries in both the hospital and field settings.[13] As emergency medicine evolved, many of the methods (e.g., resuscitation) and techniques (e.g., emergency ultrasound) applied in the emergency department have been adapted to and utilized in disaster settings. Similarly, military medical experience in warfare has both benefited from participation by emergency medical professionals[14] and provided insights, techniques, and experience that has advanced medical care in conflict and nonconflict disaster response.[15]

Across all organization types, several important themes have emerged in modern medical and health emergency management, beyond the traditional needed to address a surge in patient volume.

## Organizational management

One of the more formal processes adopted relates to the management of organizations during an incident. The Incident Command System (ICS) was developed by firefighting professionals in the 1980s through FIRESCOPE.[16] A rough adaptation was promulgated for use by hospitals in the 1980s: the Hospital Emergency Incident Command System (HEICS). This was replaced by improved guidance, Hospital Incident Command System (HICS), for hospitals to manage emergency response.[17] The Department of Veterans Affairs (VA) developed a more operationally oriented incident management approach and influenced the revision of HICS. The VA also funded a more comprehensive training curriculum (developed by this chapter's authors), designed to be applicable to any hospital, not just VA medical centers.[18] A post 9/11 2003 White House directive (Homeland Security Presidential Directive 5) compelled all domestic emergency response organizations, including public health organizations across the country and the Centers for Disease Control and Prevention, to adapt response management methodologies consistent with ICS.[19]

## Conceptual relationship between "disaster medicine" and "medical and health emergency management"

While Disaster Medicine has focused primarily upon patient care in emergency and disaster settings, Medical and Health Emergency Management has focused upon management systems, continuity of operations, and the critical support services for the practice of disaster medicine. Fortunately, health care professionals led by emergency medical and emergency nursing staff have increasingly recognized that successful application of disaster medicine in either the hospital or field settings requires a solid foundation addressed by these management principles. Similar concepts apply to conducting public health activities such as mass prophylaxis or complex rapid epidemiology.

## Enhancement of public health *and* health care services continuity through the interrelationship of public health and health care services emergency management

An increasing recognition of the interconnectedness of public health and health care is currently underway across the United States, particularly in the areas of emergency health care delivery and continuity of health care services. The painful lessons experienced by New Orleans hospitals and long-term care facilities in the aftermath of the 2005 Hurricane Katrina demonstrated the tragedy when health care systems fail. It also illustrated that when private health care services fail, the situation becomes a public health emergency with jurisdictional responsibility falling to the local government and its public health agency. This raised national awareness for emergency public health officials to develop capability to assist health care organizations in sustaining and/or rapidly recovering health care operations. It also increased recognition of the importance of promoting mitigation measures in public health and health care systems to reduce the probability and the consequences of future health care system failures. This important and professional management mission has been reinforced by more recent incidents, including the 2012 Hurricane Sandy impact on the New York–New Jersey communities which caused flooding and utility failures in large hospitals and prompted multiple emergency evacuations.[20] These incidents re-emphasize that mitigation measures to reduce risk from likely hazards are critically important and must be defined, planned, and completed in a timely manner.

### Specialty health care services and medical surge

The past 15 years also witnessed the recognition that mass casualties may not be primarily the typical blunt trauma experienced in mass transportation mishaps. The specter of mass chemical casualties similar to or worse than the 1995 Tokyo Sarin attack prompted the development of effective and rapidly available decontamination facilities for chemically contaminated patients.[21] Because patient arrival would be through the emergency department, much of this development was prompted by emergency medicine physicians and nurses. Other unusual casualty incidents have illustrated specialty situations requiring specific emergency care capabilities:

- Mass burn casualties, prompted by experiences such as the Rhode Island nightclub fire;[22]
- Highly publicized mass shootings, such as the Virginia Tech and other campus shootings, demonstrated mass penetrating injury situations; and
- SARS and pandemic influenza raised the specter of mass pulmonary illness.

Health care organizations and public health have recognized incidents like these as risks in their own communities, and have begun planning and preparedness to manage and respond to them.

### Evolution of emergency concepts and terminology

The National Incident Management System (NIMS), issued by the US Department of Homeland Security in 2004 and revised in 2008[23] made the use of standardized terminology and response concepts a requirement for federal preparedness funding. Public health and health care organizations were prompted to adopt the ICS methods referenced above in a more formal and widespread fashion. Importantly, NIMS describes not only Incident Management Teams for direct management of the impacts of an incident but also describes Multiagency Coordination Systems (MACS). The latter entity coordinates across a jurisdiction's agencies (jurisdictional emergency operations centers), within a large department such as State Public Health (department operations centers) or across divisions within a large hospital or medical center (hospital emergency operations center). These concepts have become increasingly important in effective public health and health care emergency response and are becoming more refined.

### Interaction as part of a broader health care system

As health care organizations began conversing with each other, concepts evolved (many based on MACS activities) to provide a framework for interfacing across organizations and the multiple levels of government. A project funded by Department of Health and Human Services (DHHS) produced the Medical Surge Capacity and Capability (MSCC) manual,[24] which focused on a multilayered strategy for:
- Managing coordination within each individual health care facility (Tier 1);
- Interfacing with geographically proximate health care facilities and with public health and other local agencies (Tiers 2 and 3); and
- Coordinating with regional, statewide, interstate regional, and federal capabilities (Tiers 4, 5 6) (Figure 9.1).

This has been adopted by the US DHHS Hospital Preparedness Program[25] as a central organizing strategy for federally funded health care preparedness. As a result of this guidance, many health care organizations began planning not just *preparedness*, but actual *response* actions together. It is concerning, however, that many may not be realizing the full potential by expanding beyond preparedness organizations such as emergency preparedness committees and regional work groups to realize the full potential of virtual organizations operating effectively under emergency response conditions (urgency, uncertainty, and high stakes). A follow-on MSCC manual funded by DHHS established more detailed guidance for how to organize and manage an EHC specifically under response conditions, describing an EHC Healthcare Coalition Response Team (HCRT) and its concept of operations.[26] Ultimately, EHCs have been implemented in multiple jurisdictions such as Kings County, WA, and Washington DC, with effective interface and cooperation between the health care coalitions and the jurisdiction's public health and other emergency-related authorities.

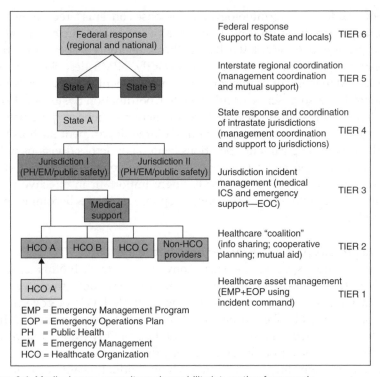

**Figure 9.1** Medical surge capacity and capability integration framework

Health care facility evacuation, mutual aid, and other key capabilities have been addressed through EHCs, driven by emergency health care professionals.

### Interface between public health and emergency health care delivery during rapidly evolving emergencies

A critical component of the above described systems is the interface between health care organizations and public health (facilitated by the MSCC Tier 2 health care coalitions). The anthrax 2001 incident in the National Capital Region highlighted the importance of effective emergency health care connectedness to local, state, and national public health. In this incident, the impact of the anthrax letters in the National Capital Area was rapidly evolving with decision to provide prophylaxis for exposure based entirely on new data discovered daily about the locations of potential exposure for patients. Given the rapid pace of this evolving emergency, situation updates were assembled by the health care facilities and the Office of the US Capitol Attending Physician (which was the health care capability with the best understanding of the health risks) and then shared with local and state public health as well as other health care organizations. This type of real-time two-way information sharing has evolved in many jurisdictions to promote a better common operating picture across public health and health care organizations.

Over the past decade since 9/11 and the 2001 anthrax dissemination, public health has also increasingly adopted modern emergency management principles and processes for before, during, and after disaster response. This has improved the ability of public health and health care organizations to interface during preparedness as well as emergency response and recovery.

## Medical response teams

Historically, emergency medicine concepts were adapted for, and in large part shaped, organizations that provide advanced medical care in the field, such as the US National Disaster Medical System's Disaster Medical Assistance Teams (DMATs), international field medical teams (e.g., nongovernmental organizations such as International Medical Corps[27]), and operational medicine teams (e.g., Urban Search and Rescue and Law Enforcement Tactical Teams). Emergency medicine physicians and paramedics established early sophisticated pre-hospital medical care teams for unusual nonhospital environments such as deep mines, caves, and structural failures,[28] and widespread earthquake building collapse,[29] tactical law enforcement support,[30] and Urban Search and Rescue Medical Teams.[31]

DMATs[32] were first developed in the 1980s as part of the National Disaster Medical System managed by DHHS in partnership with the Federal Emergency Management Agency (FEMA), VA, and the Department of Defense.[33] The first deployments of these teams occurred in 1989 to disasters in the United States and its territories.[34] Emergency physicians, emergency nurses, and paramedicine professionals were prominent leaders on the first DMATs that reached deployment status for DHHS.

During the same 1980s timeframe, the confined space medical team concepts developed by specialized medical response team (SMRT) were extended to define the collapsed structure medical team as an integral element of the Urban Search and Rescue (US&R) task force, both through the Office of US Foreign Disaster Assistance and FEMA. This development was led by emergency physicians and paramedics and advanced the application of emergency medicine and emergency care practice to the austere environment of collapsed structures and entrapped patients in confined spaces.[35] The concepts were later extended by California emergency care professionals to swift water rescue and other emergency response capabilities.

It is interesting to note that at large-scale disaster sites, such as the 1995 Oklahoma City bombing and the 9/11 crash sites at the Pentagon, it was primarily emergency medicine providers from the FEMA US&R that provided public health and preventive medicine oversight of the emergency workers during the extended emergency response period (along with military medicine professionals at the 9/11 Pentagon site) as there was little direct public health oversight. Increasingly, public health officials have recognized they too have a significant field disaster role assisting with safety and public health risk assessments, and many public health departments are preparing to provide services within active disaster sites.

## Future

Emergency care professionals are poised to take on increased relevance in the future of emergency and disaster response. Public health and health care system leaders are recognizing that future medical and public health emergencies may present far more casualties than can be effectively managed using day-to-day service delivery with currently available resources. Many of the issues are being discussed within the framework of "Altered" or "Crisis Standards of Care,"[36] but this approach has encountered political, ethical, and operational roadblocks that raise major doubts as to feasibility of this approach. An approach more consistent with emergency management may be indicated.

Much of the activity in public health and health care preparedness over the past decade has focused almost exclusively on "preparedness." Achieving true readiness for emergencies and disasters requires a much more focused effort on defining the specific response models for use during emergencies, followed by response-oriented guidance that will work in the projected no-notice, sudden onset, uncertain environment of a major incident. For example, the HCRT was described in the MSCC as the organization that will facilitate coalition member organizations' emergency actions and facilitate the interface with local government partners, including public health. Position descriptions for HCRT, along with operational checklists and other tools have demonstrated effectiveness for both operational level training and HCRT response performance in multiple emergencies in Washington DC. Preparing towards this model, and other realistic response models, will produce actual readiness.

A more consistent approach to standard incident management within health care facilities is needed, along with better defined and effective emergency operations centers to coordinate the many divisions and facilities in large hospitals and medical centers. This may be addressed and the guidance memorialized in more useful emergency operations plans that include rapidly available tools such as operational checklists for key response positions, forms that drive proactive incident action planning, and special considerations for unusual hazard situations. This is particularly important for major threats to maintaining a medically safe and secure physical environment (from utility compromise, contaminated or contagious arriving patients, terrorism, or other threats of violence).

A new version of the HICS is under development and may assist with this important issue.

Emergency medicine's approach to major incidents can serve as a model for a newly evolving discipline – Emergency Public Health. Just as the birth of emergency medicine occurred in the 1970s and 1980s because traditional medical specialties were not meeting the needs of the public for emergency health care, it is becoming clear that Emergency Public Health is needed as a defined public health discipline that addresses public health science using strategy and methods drawn from emergency management, incident response, and emergency medicine. This goes well beyond the current approach of using traditional public health institutions, with public health emergency preparedness[37] layered on top. Emergency Public Health must become proficient in major complex emergency responses across the broad range of hazards in which public health can have a key role. Relevant concepts include operational information management, strategic and tactical decision making under uncertainty, and appropriate resource utilization in challenging situations. These capabilities within a public health organization will enhance the ability for all the specialty areas (e.g., epidemiology, public health laboratories, public information, mass prophylaxis) to perform optimally in complex incidents. Many additional mitigation and preparedness concepts may translate easily from emergency management and emergency medicine to the public health domain.

As the nation evolves its mitigation and preparedness efforts while enhancing efficiency and effectiveness, the recently developed concept of MSCC EHCs will become more prominent. These platforms adapt processes and procedures from emergency management and emergency medical systems. They serve as facilitators of effective response for both acute care medical organizations and public health alike, with emergency care professionals commonly serving at the interface positions, and provide a far deeper capability and capacity than individual organizations. The EHC provides an effective platform for establishing mutual aid and cooperative assistance mechanisms to bring medical resources rapidly to the points of medical needs, rather than trying to stockpile large numbers of resources at each facility's location or futilely trying to distribute mass casualties evenly from a large uncontrolled scene.

The capabilities needed to enhance and sustain continuity of operations in health care facilities, with the benefit of the health care coalition processes, may be the most compelling reason for every health care organization to enroll in a response-effective EHC. The practice of establishing a robust coalition-level hazard vulnerability analysis to provide an informed basis for consensus on the greatest risks at the coalition and community level, and then planning and establishing cost effective risk reduction initiatives, will continue to spread. As federal funding for public health and health care emergency preparedness decreases, it is important that coalition capabilities and partnership with public health be maintained through lean mechanisms that, once established, can be sustained with minimal external funding. Demonstrating risk reduction for participating organizations may also prompt wider acceptance of voluntary funding from coalition member organizations.

Public health has begun to establish similar coalition-type relationships between local public health jurisdictions, and this is being encouraged through a Centers for Disease Control and Prevention-sponsored Risk Based Funding Program that looks at public health risk at the regional level of a metropolitan statistical area rather than just intrastate regions.[38] Public health coalitions at a metropolitan regional level may be critical in the future in achieving public health surge capacity and extending public health capabilities across even rural jurisdictions where rudimentary or absent local public health elements currently exist.

## References

1 The Joint Commission web site. Available at: http://www.jointcommission.org/ (accessed 30 November 2013).
2 Okimura T, Kouichiro S, Fukuda A, Kohama A, Takasu N, Ishimatsu S, et al. Tokyo subway sarin attack, Part 1: Community emergency response. Acad Emerg Med. 1998;5:613–7.
3 Hogan DE, Waeckerle JF, Dire DJ, Lillibridge SR. Emergency department impact of the Oklahoma City terrorist bombing. Ann Emerg Med. 1999;34:160–7.
4 US Government Accountability Office. Combating terrorism: observations on the nunn-lugar-domenici domestic preparedness program. 1986. Available at: http://www.gao.gov/products/T-NSIAD-99-16 (accessed 30 November 2013).
5 Office of the Assistant Secretary for Preparedness and Response. Hospital preparedness program overview: FY02 to present and beyond. Available at: http://www.phe.gov/Preparedness/planning/hpp/Pages/overview.aspx (accessed 30 November 2013).
6 Gray BH, Hebert K. Hospitals in Hurricane Katrina: challenges facing custodial institutions in a disaster. J Health Care Poor Underserved. 2007;18(2):283–98.
7 VHA Office of Emergency Management. VHA Office of Emergency Management: comprehensive emergency management (CEMP). Available at: http://www.va.gov/VHAEMERGENCYMANAGEMENT/CEMP/VHA_OEM_CEMP_Main.asp (accessed 30 November 2013).
8 George Washington University. Healthcare Emergency Management Competencies, Curriculum and Certification Recommendations developed under contract for the Veterans Health Affairs. 2010. Available at: http://www.gwu.edu/~icdrm/projects/VHA2/index.htm#download (accessed 30 November 2013).
9 Federal Emergency Management Agency. CPG 101: comprehensive preparedness guide developing and maintaining emergency operations plans. 2010. Available at: http://www.fema.gov/library/viewRecord.do?=&id=5697 (accessed 30 November 2013).

10 Centers for Medicare and Medicaid Services . Survey and certification: emergency preparedness for every emergency. Available at: http://www.cms.gov/Medicare /Provider-Enrollment-and-Certification/SurveyCertEmergPrep/Downloads /SandC_EPChecklist_Provider.pdf (accessed 30 November 2013).

11 World Association for Disaster and Emergency Medicine (WADEM). History. Available at: http://www.wadem.org/mission.html (accessed 30 November 2013).

12 American College of Emergency Physicians. History of ACEP. Available at: http://www.acep.org/aboutus/history/ (accessed 30 November 2013).

13 Gans L, Kennedy T. Management of unique clinical entities in disaster medicine. Emerg Med Clin North Am. 1996;14(2):301–26.

14 Burkle FM, Orebaugh S, Barendse BR. Emergency medicine in the Persian Gulf War – Part 1: preparations for triage and combat casualty care. Ann Emerg Med. 1994;23:742–9.

15 Grisson TE, Farmer JC. The provision of sophisticated critical care beyond the hospital: lessons from physiology and military experiences that apply to civil disaster medical response. Critical Care Med. 2005;33(1):S13–21.

16 Stambler KS, Barbera JA. Engineering the incident command and multiagency coordination systems. J Homeland Security Emerg Manage 2011;8(1):Art. 43.

17 Hospital Incident Command System Guidebook. California Emergency Medical Services Authority (EMSA). 2006. Available at: http://www .emsa.ca.gov/disaster/default.asp (accessed 30 November 2013).

18 George Washington University. Healthcare emergency management competencies, curriculum and certification recommendations developed under contract for the Veterans Health Affairs. (2010) Available at: http://www.gwu.edu /~icdrm/projects/VHA2/index.htm#download (accessed 30 November 2013).

19 Homeland Security Presidential Directive 5: Management of Domestic Incidents. The White House, 2003.

20 Teperman S. Hurricane Sandy and the greater New York health care system. J Trauma Acute Care Surg. 2013;74(6):1401–10.

21 MacIntyre AG, Christopher GW, Eitzen E Jr,, Gum R, Weir S, DeAtley C, et al. Weapons of mass destruction events with contaminated casualties: effective planning for health care facilities. J Am Med Assoc. 2000;283(2):242–9.

22 Dacey MJ. Tragedy and response: the Rhode Island nightclub fire. New Engl J Med. 2003;349(21):1990–2.

23 Federal Emergency Management Agency. National Incident Management System. 2008. Available at: http://www.fema.gov/pdf/emergency/nims/NIMS_core.pdf (accessed 30 November 2013).

24 Barbera JA, MacIntyre AG, (Knebel A, Trabert E, eds). Medical Surge Capacity and Capability: A Management System for Integrating Medical and Health Resources During Large-Scale Emergencies, 2nd ed. 2007. Available at: http://www.phe.gov/Preparedness/planning/mscc/handbook/Documents /mscc080626.pdf (accessed 20 December 2013).

25 Hospital Preparedness program (HPP). Available at: http://www.phe.gov /Preparedness/planning/hpp/Pages/default.aspx (accessed 20 November 2013).

26 Barbera JA, MacIntyre AG. (Knebel A, Trabert E, eds). (2009) Medical surge capacity and capability: the MSCC healthcare coalition in emergency response and recovery. Available at: http://www.phe.gov/Preparedness /planning/mscc/healthcarecoalition/Pages/default.aspx (accessed 20 December 2013).

27 Simon RR, Hyman MH. Establishing underground medical clinics in rural Afghanistan: the International Medical Corps experience. Ann Intern Med. 1988;108:477–80.

28 Kunkle RF. Emergency medical care in the underground environment. Prehosp Disaster Med. 1986;2(1–4):54–5.

29 Moede JD. The dynamics of medical care for structural collapse victims. In: The Hidden Disaster: Urban Search and Rescue. San Diego, CA: JEMS Publishing Company, 1989: pp. 109–19.

30 Schwartz RB, McManus JG, Swienton RE. Forward. In: Tactical Emergency Medicine. Philadelphia, PA: Lippencott Williams & Wilkins, 2008.

31 Barbera JA, Cadoux CG. Search, rescue and evacuation. In: Critical Care Clinics: Disaster Management 7, 1991: pp. 321–37.

32 Disaster Medical Assistance Team (DMAT). Public Health Emergency Preparedness. Available at: http://www.phe.gov/Preparedness/responders/ndms /teams/Pages/dmat.aspx (accessed 7 November 2013).

33 Franco C, Toner E, Waldhorn R, Inglesby TV, O'Toole T. The national disaster medical system: past, present, and suggestions for the future. Biosecurity Bioterrorism 2007;5(4):319–25.

34 Roth PB, Vogel A, Key G, Hall D, Stockhoff CT. The St Croix disaster and the national disaster medical system. Ann Emerg Med. 1991;20(4):391–5.

35 Barbera JA, Lozano M. Urban search and rescue medical teams: FEMA task force system. Prehosp. Disaster Med. 1993;8(4):349–55.

36 National Academies of Science-Institute of Medicine, Board on Health Science Policy. Crisis Standards of Care: A Systems Framework for Catastrophic Disaster Response. 2012. Available at: http://www.iom.edu/Reports /2012/Crisis-Standards-of-Care-A-Systems-Framework-for-Catastrophic-Disaster -Response.aspx (accessed 30 November 2013).

37 Nelson C, Lurie N, Wasserman E, Zakowski S, Leuschner KJ. Conceptualizing and defining public health emergency preparedness. RAND (working paper May 2008). Available at: http://www.rand.org/content/dam /rand/pubs/working_papers/2008/RAND_WR543.pdf (accessed 30 November 2013).

38 Department of Health and Human Services Centers for Disease Control and Prevention. Fiscal Year 2011 RFA/PFA Number: CCD-RFA-TP11-1101cont11. 2013. Available at: http://www.cdc.gov/phpr/documents/PHEP_FY_2011.pdf (accessed 30 November 2013).

# CHAPTER 10

# Emergency public health

## Rebecca Katz[1], Anthony Macintyre[2], and Joseph Barbera[2,3,4]

[1]Emergency Medicine and Health Policy, The George Washington University, USA
[2]Department of Emergency Medicine, The George Washington University, USA
[3]Engineering Management (Crisis and Emergency Management), The George Washington University, USA
[4]Institute for Crisis, Disaster, and Risk Management, Department of Engineering Management and Systems Engineering The George Washington University, USA

## Introduction

The anthrax dissemination incident of 2001, the novel SARS outbreak in 2003, and the more recent 2009 H1N1 influenza pandemic all had two things in common:

1 They required significant public health input to, and management of the emergency response; and

2 Despite their significant impacts, they could each have been much worse if a few hazard characteristics had been slightly different (e.g., more effective delivery mechanisms – anthrax; enhanced contagiousness – SARS).

The resultant question may be posed: is public health (at all levels of government) poised to respond to more unusual, dynamic, and uncertain incidents that have the potential for far greater morbidity and mortality?

The role of public health in emergencies, as part of the larger response effort, or as the lead discipline, has been difficult to characterize. In one instance, public health *preparedness* has been defined as having the capacities, plans, and procedures in place to detect, respond, and recover from acute public health emergencies that have the capacity to overwhelm routine capabilities.[1] How this translates to measurable effective public health emergency *response* remains somewhat elusive.

*Emergency Care and The Public's Health*, First Edition.
Edited by Jesse M. Pines, Jameel Abualenain, James Scott and Robert Shesser.
© 2014 John Wiley & Sons, Ltd. Published 2014 by John Wiley & Sons, Ltd.

## Public health functions during response to an emergency

Trust for America's Health identifies two broad functional requirements for public health during emergencies:
1 Supporting basic functions of a public health system; and
2 Having the training, procedures, leadership, laws and regulations, and plans in place for broad cooperation and execution of mitigation strategies to address public health emergencies.[2]

These concepts can be equated to the continuity missions and surge missions described in the previous chapter in reference to health care emergency management.[3] In other words, the response and/or recovery requirements of public health organizations can be framed as:

1. *Public health continuity of operations.* Maintain regular operations despite hazard impact on the organization, including assurance of personnel safety.

2. *Public health surge capacity.* Increase the frequency or pace of regular operations to meet the increase in public health service delivery.

3. *Public health surge capability.* Address unique or unusual hazards and the resultant specialized public health needs, which may pose a significant threat to the health or well-being of a community.

4. *Public health recovery.* Manage rapid return to normal operations, specifically addressing backlogs in critical public health and health care services and facilitating return-to-readiness of public health emergency response resources.

A further delineation of public health functions within this context helps define exactly what public health must achieve during emergencies and may provide context for a potential new sub-discipline, that of emergency public health.

## Basic functions of public health

Similar to the health care industry, there is an expectation that the public health sector will maintain its day-to-day operations during emergencies and disasters. Before considering additional emergency activities that public health may be called upon to perform, the capability to continue important day-to-day public health functions must be addressed (Box 10.1). These should be examined within the context of continuity of operations.

---

**Box 10.1 Essential public health services**

The Essential Services provide a working definition of public health and a guiding framework for the responsibilities of local public health systems:[5]

- Monitor health status to identify and solve community health problems
- Diagnose and investigate health problems and health hazards in the community

- Inform, educate, and empower people about health issues
- Mobilize community partnerships and action to identify and solve health problems
- Develop policies and plans that support individual and community health efforts
- Enforce laws and regulations that protect health and ensure safety
- Link people to needed personal health services and assure the provision of health care when otherwise unavailable
- Assure competent public and personal health care workforce
- Evaluate effectiveness, accessibility, and quality of personal and population-based health services
- Research for new insights and innovative solutions to health problems

The essential public health services described in Box 10.1 speak to the broad range of activities supported by the public health infrastructure, which can range from community, state, tribal, and federal level public health departments, to laboratory networks used for surveillance and diagnostics, to academic facilities, and private entities supporting the public health mission. The broad range of activities and expertise associated with public health is best illustrated through the concentrations offered in most public health schools, which include policy, management, environmental health, global health, epidemiology (including chronic disease, infectious disease, and nosocomial illness), biostatistics, community and preventive health, reproductive health/maternal and child health, health communications/risk communications, exercise science, nutrition, and social and behavioral health. Along with these areas of expertise and sub-disciplines, the public health community focuses these disciplines and services in critical areas of need that may include obesity, HIV/AIDS, biosurveillance, cancer, electronic health records, and health insurance. Emergency public health, or the ability of the public health community to manage the detection, assessment, response, and recovery to an acute emergency, is just one responsibility, and one that has not traditionally received specific academic attention.

## Emergency functions of public health

The roles of public health during emergency response can be viewed as extensions of the above baseline functions (equivalent to surge capacity) or can entail very specialized surge capabilities. Examples of potential public health emergency functions include the following (all of the items with asterisks are consistent with the Public Health Emergency Preparedness [PHEP] core capabilities published by the CDC as guidance for their PHEP program):

- Surge capacity
  - Increased volume of public messaging for general and agent-specific population guidance*
  - Enhanced and time-compressed epidemiologic activities*
  - Increased frequency of diagnostic testing (such as through regional or national public health laboratories and environmental laboratories)*
  - Increased advisory support to and coordination with law enforcement and other investigative and response agencies
  - Provision of care – an often overlooked fact is that public health serves in the role of primary providers of health services in some jurisdictions or for specific populations*
  - Ongoing oversight and/or support to health care organizations
- Surge capability
  - Rapid examination of anomaly situations for new pathogens or novel presentations of known pathogens, requiring unusual assessment and testing
  - Development of new diagnostic capabilities for unusual or emerging pathogens
  - Development and dissemination of guidance related to protection, diagnosis, treatment, and transmission interruption of emerging or reemerging pathogens (often this guidance may need to be conveyed initially with incomplete information)
  - Distribution of countermeasure guidance in a timely fashion to large populations*
  - Broader applications of public health law*
  - Implementation of nonpharmaceutical interventions, including school closures and other social distancing measures*
  - Development of new standards or modifications of existing ones to facilitate health care industry response
  - Others as required by the unique emergency

Though the above are emergency *response activities* that occur during incidents, it is important to note that the public health role has specific *preparedness activities* to ready itself and the community for emergencies and disasters; these differ markedly from day-to-day public health functions. A full listing of these is beyond the scope of this chapter, but many relate to system development, implementation, resource acquisition and maintenance in a ready state, personnel training, development of legal and regulatory infrastructure, and system exercise, evaluation and improvement planning. As an example, management of volunteers that may be available for emergency response (such as the Medical Reserve Corps) is conducted as a preparedness activity by public health organizations.

It is also important to note that many public health responsibilities conducted during day-to-day operations are also relevant during incident response. Biosurveillance, for example, has the potential to not only detect an anomaly but, when effectively conducted, can further characterize an incident as it evolves. A more formal definition is provided in Box 10.2.

---

**Box 10.2 Biosurveillance: Definition from National Strategy for Biosurveillance**

"The Strategy defines biosurveillance as the process of gathering, integrating, interpreting, and communicating essential information related to all-hazards threats or disease activity affecting human, animal, or plant health to achieve early detection and warning, contribute to overall situational awareness of the health aspects of an incident, and to enable better decision making at all levels."

*Source*: White House. National Strategy for Biosurveillance. July 2012

---

Various mechanisms and systems are utilized to conduct biosurveillance but many are focused only on detecting that something is happening. Few are currently robust enough to also provide the information necessary for a rapid epidemiologic investigation to determine the critical parameters of the evolving situation. All require integration with other response disciplines in order to be effective, highlighting the need for public health to integrate with the larger response architecture. The 2012 National Strategy for Biosurveillance was intended to address these issues.

## Overview of existing policies

Over the past decade, a series of polices, regulations, and legislation have been established to improve emergency preparedness and response. Though not all were developed specifically for public health, each has an impact on how emergency public health can be developed, executed, and sustained. Major legislative acts were passed starting in 2000, each adding authority and responsibility to the public health community to responsibly manage emergency events. Legislation was designed to ensure the development of medical countermeasures, prepare hospitals for surge capacity, address workforce issues, manage infectious agents, limit liabilities, and enhance biosurveillance. A series of Presidential Directives were also issued during the past decade, laying out a roadmap for biodefense strategies, response to public health and medical emergencies, life science research, and coordination of resources in preparation for and response to national emergencies. Table 10.1 is a list of selected legislation and Presidential Directives that informs and frames the following discussion on potential solutions.[6]

## Challenges

Extensive planning and policy development has advanced in the last decade. The intent was to improve public health emergency preparedness, but the volume of new guidance and direction may itself pose a challenge to public health practitioners.

There are other challenges that threaten the successful implementation of emergency public health. Perhaps one of the most significant relates to funding of our domestic public health infrastructure. Though continuity of *emergency operations* is a concern, loss of funding has implications regarding continuity of *day-to-day operations* for public health (i.e., without an emergency). Since 2001, significant federal funding has been applied to public health preparedness, yet simultaneous funding for regular public health operations is often not as robust. Many State and local health departments have challenges maintaining regular staffing. More jobs may be lost with the cessation of the Early Warning Infectious Disease Surveillance program that supported epidemiology and laboratory functions in 20 Border States. Approximately 60% of state health agencies are cutting entire programs, according to the advocacy group Trust for America's Health.[7]

Though designation of funding (often federal) for application to public health emergency capabilities is constructive, these funding mechanisms are often accompanied with administrative activities (e.g., to ensure compliance with grant mechanisms) which can be burdensome. Even if appropriately resourced, public health organizations wishing to develop emergency capabilities are confronted with a dizzying array of suggested courses of actions and priorities. No single authoritative and accepted source of guidance for emergency public health actions exists.

Another example of a significant challenge is the execution of public health law. Much of day-to-day public health activity is conducted directly by public health resources, or through laws and regulations that guide non-public health resources in conducting public health actions (e.g., reportable disease registries, sanitation guidance). A challenging function during major public health emergencies, however, is that many of the actions required for population protection and disease control may be beyond the direct authority of public health agencies. This issue was recognized in the early 2000s and potential solutions, such as the Model State Emergency Health Powers Act (MSEHPA), published in 2002, were proposed.[8] This remains an unresolved situation, as the ability to

**Table 10.1** Select emergency public health legislation and presidential directives

| Legislation | |
| --- | --- |
| Public Health Improvement Act of 2000 (Public Law 106-505) | Addresses emerging threats to the public's health and authorizes the Secretary of HHS to take appropriate response actions during a public health emergency, including investigations, treatment, and prevention |
| USA PATRIOT Act of 2001 (Public Law 107-56) | Provisions related to acquiring, handling, and transporting particularly dangerous pathogens, assistance to first responders, and funding for substantial new investments in bioterrorism preparedness and response |
| Public Health Security and Bioterrorism Preparedness and Response Act of 2002 (Public Law 107-188) | Five titles, addressing: development of medical countermeasures, creation of national disaster medical system, communications and surveillance, hospital preparedness, workforce shortages for public health emergencies, strategic nationals stockpile, control over select agents, protecting food supply, and assessing safety of water supply |
| The Project Bioshield Act of 2004 (Public Law 108-276) | Creates a guaranteed government-funded market for medical countermeasures, and included funding to purchase the products while they are still in the final stages of development |
| Public Readiness and Emergency Preparedness (PREP) Act of 2005 (Division C of the Department of Defense Emergency Supplemental Appropriations (Public Law 109-148) | Limits liability associated with public health countermeasures used on an emergency basis. The only exception is in the event of "willful misconduct" |
| Pandemic and All-Hazards Preparedness Act of 2006 (Public Law 109-417) | Adds broad provisions aimed at preparing for and responding to public health and medical emergencies, regardless of origin. PAHPA was reauthorized in 2013 |
| Implementing Recommendations of the 9/11 Commission Act of 2007 (Public Law 110-53) | Provisions pertaining preparedness grants to state and local entities, improving the incident command system, improving the sharing of intelligence information across the federal government, and the need to maintain a National Biosurveillance Integration Center |

*Continued*

**Table 10.1** (*Continued*)

*Presidential Directives, Executive Orders and Strategies*

| | |
|---|---|
| Biodefense for the twenty-first Century: National Security Presidential Directive 33/Homeland Security Presidential Directive 10, April 2004 | Strategic overview of the biological weapons threat and the Administration's approach to framing biodefense initiatives |
| Medical Countermeasures Against Weapons of Mass Destruction: Homeland Security Presidential Directive 18, February 2007 | Policies associated with medical countermeasures |
| Public Health and Medical Preparedness: Homeland Security Presidential Directive 21, October 2007 | Defines four critical components of public health and medical preparedness: robust and integrated biosurveillance system, the ability to stockpile and distribute medical countermeasures, the capacity to engage in mass casualty care in emergency situations, and building resilient communities at the state and local level |
| National Strategy for Countering Biological Threats: Presidential Policy Directive 2, November 2009 | Seven major objectives, including promoting global health security, obtaining timely and accurate insight on current and emerging risks, and transforming the international dialogue on biological threats |
| Establishing Federal Capability for the Timely Provision of Medical Countermeasures Following a Biological Attack: Executive Order 13527, December 2009 | Establishes a policy of timely provision of medical countermeasures in the event of a biological attack and tasks the federal government with assisting state and local entities in this endeavor. The order also spells out the role of the US Postal Service in the delivery of medical countermeasures and calls on HHS to develop continuity of operations plans in the event of a large-scale biological attack |
| National Preparedness Presidential Policy Directive 8, March 2011 | Requires the development of a national preparedness goal and the creation of a National Preparedness System to integrate guidance, programs, and processes to build and sustain capabilities essential for preparedness |

practically implement controversial sections of MSEHPA has been openly questioned.[9] For example, a single-sided approach of public health directing health care resources, as suggested in MSEHPA, is unlikely to be a workable solution. Concerns about other large-scale public health measures are supported by past experiences from actual incidents.[10]

The ability of infections to cross borders (intranational and international) and rapidly spread beyond the traditional epidemiologic patterns provides another set of challenges for emergency public health. Advances in technology have provided the ability to recognize a new or re-emerging disease rapidly. But it is the sheer speed of spread of dangerous disease or contamination that may be the greatest challenge, especially for public health threats with a surreptitious onset. Earliest possible recognition, rapid epidemiologic investigation to characterize the threat, and establishing the confidence, authority, and public trust to rapidly make high commitment response decisions are critical. The ability to effect multidisciplinary response actions to implement public health decisions also must be assured. Differing management systems, public health laws, and information requirements pose complexities that are not easily resolved, though significant achievements have been made.[11,12] Cross border collaboration in the international arena has expanded with attention to the building of host country capacities such as has been done under the International Health Regulations (2005). The collaboration in recognizing a new and potentially severe corona virus, its rapid DNA sequencing and expedient development and dissemination of diagnostic testing has demonstrated the impressive technological advances in recent years, and the ability of public health researchers and managers to work together once an emergency situation is recognized.[13]

There are also challenges associated with the deployment of public health personnel into the field across borders with further attention needed on addressing liabilities and the establishment of agreements before an incident occurs (whether bilaterally or multilaterally). This also applies to the sharing of medical countermeasures.

## Emergency public health as a defined discipline

The complexity of functions that public health must perform during emergencies, the architecture of legislation over the past decade, and the challenges posed argue for the development and maintenance of a new discipline within public health: emergency public health. A discipline can be defined in different ways, but recurring themes include the following:[14]

- Common body of knowledge;
- Common body of research;

- Common terminology;
- Agreed upon competencies;
- Recognized study curriculum; and
- Accreditation process.

This is not an easy or rapid undertaking and one that requires allocation of funding. In addition, coordination with multiple bodies (e.g., Association of Schools and Programs of Public Health, ASPPH) would be required in the development and maintenance of such a system.

Defining a discipline, as a first step, may seem esoteric but in reality has tremendous implications for achieving professional recognition; defining overarching goals and objectives of the discipline is a critical element in this definition. Only then can core tenets of the discipline be defined. A recently proposed definition for health care emergency management is worth examining for potential adaptation: "Healthcare emergency management is the science of managing complex systems and multidisciplinary personnel to address emergencies and disasters in healthcare systems across all hazards and through the phases of mitigation, preparedness, response, and recovery."[14]

Several unifying principles can be considered as overarching guidance in establishing this prospective discipline. As many of these concepts are well integrated into other response disciplines (e.g., emergency management, emergency medicine), they may serve to not only enhance public health response activities, but may also enhance integration with other response efforts:

- The concepts inherent in an "all hazards" approach should serve as central doctrine. Both health and medical organizations have often focused on individual specific hazards. Greater efficiencies can be realized by prioritizing program issues applicable across hazards and then secondarily focusing on individual issues. As an example, a response plan should be written to address commonalities in any emergency, then individual hazard issues addressed in smaller attachments to the overarching plan.
- Emergency Public Health should consider doctrine from other response disciplines. As an example, NFPA 1600 (Standard on Disaster/Emergency Management and Business Continuity Programs) is a standard that establishes a well-recognized and validated framework for organizations to follow during preparedness *and* response. Another example can be found in FEMA's Comprehensive Planning Guide 101 which includes, among other things, guidance on the format of an Emergency Operations Plan (EOP – Disaster Plan).[15]
- Both medicine and health have historical experience attempting to manage emergency response with preparedness organizations such as committees or other everyday management mechanisms. Preparedness

organizations include structures and methodologies that are necessarily designed to address regulatory and other slower deliberate processes. For example, committees that debate different approaches with an opportunity for all voices to contribute are a common example. These approaches are often insufficient given the time urgency or lack of resources available during response. Different approaches are necessary as outlined in and advocated by the implementation of Incident Command System (ICS)/National Incident Management System (NIMS).

• During preparedness, a priority should be placed on addressing basic capabilities and those that are achievable. Intellectually challenging topics that are complex and less likely to be encountered (though still high impact) can distract preparedness resources before these more basic capabilities have been addressed. As an example, an organization might consider prioritizing basic functions such as information management methodologies before considering the complexities inherent with the allocation of scarce resources, which in some instances, may require legislative changes.[16]

• Performance measurements systems are well researched and provide mechanisms to improve organizational capabilities. Already in existence for day-to-day functions, further adaptation for emergency preparedness and response should occur.

The adaptation of these principles may lead to innovative solutions to the many challenges, only some of which have been listed in this chapter.

## Conclusions

Public health, as a broad discipline, is responsible for many of the advancements in modern society. As with other disciplines, however, alternate approaches have become necessary over the past two decades to address emerging threats and to enhance emergency response to already recognized hazards. New approaches to management of complex systems, information management, and prioritization of efforts are necessary and can be enhanced through the adaptation of concepts from other response disciplines. These concepts could serve not only to improve the execution of emergency public health functions, but also to increase the integration of efforts with these other emergency response disciplines.

## References

1  Nelson C, Lurie N, Wasserman J, Zakowski S. Conceptulaizing and defining public health emergency preparedness. Am J Public Health. 2007;97(S1):S9–11.
2  Trust for America's Health. Ready or Not? Protecting the Public's Health from Diseases, Disasters, and Bioterrorism. Available at: http://www.tfah.org/assets/files/TFAH2011ReadyorNot_09.pdf (accessed 30 November 2013).

3 MacIntyre A, Barbera J, Brewster P. Health care emergency management: establishing the science of managing mass casualty and mass effect incidents. Disaster Med Public Health Prep 2009;3:S52–8.

4 World Health Organization. Global Alert and Response. Severe Acute Respiratory Syndrome (SARS). Available at: http://www.who.int/csr/sars/en/ (accessed 30 November 2013).

5 National Public Health Performance Standards Program (NPHPSP). 10 essential public health services. Available at: http://www.cdc.gov/nphpsp/essentialservices.html (accessed 30 November 2013).

6 Portions of this section are drawn from Katz R. Public health preparedness. In: Teitlebaum J, Wilensky SE (eds). Essentials of Public Health: Health Policy and the Law, 2nd edition. Jones and Bartlett, 2012.

7 Trust for America's Health. (2011) Investing in America's Health. Available at: http://www.healthyamericans.org/assets/files/Investing%20in%20America's%20Health.pdf (accessed 30 November 2013).

8 Lawrence O, Gostin JW, Sapsin SP, Teret SB, Burris S, Mair JS, et al. The model state emergency powers act: planning for and response to bioterrorism and naturally occurring infectious diseases. J Am Med Assoc. 2002;288(5):622–8.

9 Richards E, Rathbun K. Legislative alternatives to the model state emergency health powers act (MSEHPA). LSU Program in Law, Science, and Public Health White Paper #2. 2003.

10 Barbera J, MacIntyre A, Gostin L, Inglesby T, O'Toole T, DeAtley C, et al. Large-scale quarantine following biological terrorism in the United States: scientific examination, logistics, and legal limits and possible consequences. J Am Med Assoc. 2001;286(21):2711–7.

11 Centers for Disease Control and prevention (CDC). Early Warning Infectious Disease Surveillance (EWIDS) Program Activities on the Northern and Southern Border States. Available at: http://www.bt.cdc.gov/surveillance/ewids/ (accessed 30 November 2013).

12 North American Plan for Animal and Pandemic Influenza. 2012. Available at: http://www.phe.gov/Preparedness/international/Documents/napapi.pdf (accessed 30 November 2013).

13 International Society for Infectious Diseases. ProMED-mail. (2012) Novel Coronavirus – Saudi Arabia (13): History, Collateral Damage. Available at: http://www.promedmail.org/direct.php?id=20121021.1356623 (accessed 30 November 2013).

14 MacIntyre A, Barbera J, Brewster P. Health care emergency management: establishing the science of managing mass casualty and mass effect incidents. Disaster Med Public Health Prep. 2009;3:S52–8.

15 Federal Emergency Management Agency. Comprehensive Preparedness Guide 101 (CPG 101). Washington DC. (2010) Available at: http://www.fema.gov/pdf/about/divisions/npd/CPG_101_V2.pdf (accessed 30 November 2013).

16 Hanfling D, Altevogt B, Viswanathan K, Gostin LO. Crisis Standards of Care: A Systems Framework For Catastrophic Disaster Response. Washington DC: National Academies Press, 2012.

# PART 5

# Emergency care payment reform and legal issues

# The role of the emergency department in care coordination

**Emily R. Carrier**
*Center for Studying Health System Change, USA*

## Introduction

Emergency care may appear to be a series of isolated provider–patient interactions involving little or no interaction with other providers or elements of the health care system. In fact, care coordination is important for high-quality emergency care and consumes significant amounts of emergency provider time.

Care coordination in emergency departments (ED) occurs at three levels:
- *Within EDs*. ED providers coordinate with each other, both on teams working together and at change of shift when one provider or team hands off care to another.
- *Within hospitals*. ED providers coordinate care with other hospital-based physicians, and other services such as social service, case management, etc.
- *Within communities*. ED providers coordinate care with community-based physicians to share information about patients and to ensure a safe disposition.

This chapter briefly discusses best practices in ED team-based care and handoffs, but the primary focus is coordination of care with community-based physicians.

## Importance of care coordination

Care fragmentation is defined as receiving non-coordinated care from many different providers and affects every phase of health care delivery. Care fragmentation is also associated with increased utilization and costs.[1] ED providers may contribute to fragmentation through their actions, or

*Emergency Care and The Public's Health*, First Edition.
Edited by Jesse M. Pines, Jameel Abualenain, James Scott and Robert Shesser.
© 2014 John Wiley & Sons, Ltd. Published 2014 by John Wiley & Sons, Ltd.

may find themselves dealing with the consequences of fragmentation caused by others. Care continuity, "the relationship between a single practitioner and a patient that extends beyond specific episodes of illness or disease"[2] is the converse of care fragmentation. Saultz[3] and others describe three forms of continuity of care:

1 In *longitudinal continuity*, the patient's usual source of care is a single geographic location.

2 In *informational continuity*, all of the patient's caregivers share a common medical record.

3 In *interpersonal continuity*, a single individual provides most or all of a patient's care.

Many patients with existing longitudinal relationships may still experience care discontinuities. For example, a patient's care may be divided between a primary care physician (PCP) and a specialist working in separate independent practices who rarely communicate with each other and do not share a common record. ED visits may add to a patient's discontinuity if the ED record is not seamlessly merged with the patient's longitudinal care records.

Care coordination has been defined as "a function that helps ensure that the patient's needs and preferences for health services and information sharing across people, functions and sites are met over time. Coordination maximizes the value of services delivered to patients by facilitating beneficial, efficient, safe and high-quality patient experiences and improved healthcare outcomes."[4] By encouraging the development of hospital systems that support care coordination, providers can reduce any additional fragmentation resulting from their ED care. By sharing information with other providers, emergency physicians can avoid gaps or duplication in care, ensure that patients obtain needed follow-up, address utilization issues, and perform specific tasks such as medication reconciliation.

There is no quantitative way to measure coordination and little "best practices" guidance as to which kinds of efforts are the most effective. Formal study and development of care coordination in the ED is just beginning, and will certainly become more important over the coming years. The Transitions of Care Committee, a group made up of specialty societies representing general internists, hospitalists, and ED physicians which outlines broad principles of coordination around care transitions such as accountability and timely feedback of information, states that "the emergency department represents a unique subset of transitions of care" and that the broad range of acuity and needs ED patients experience "precludes a single approach to ED transitions of care coordination."[5] The Centers for Medicare and Medicaid Services Meaningful Use Menu

Set Measures called for participating hospitals to provide patients or receiving providers with a summary care record for at least 50% of care transitions, which may include ED discharges.[6]

## Current literature on care coordination in the ED

There have been several observational studies of teamwork both within the ED, and between EDs and other hospital services. There has been very little research on coordination of care between EDs and other settings in the community. This is in part due to the challenges of conducting research across different care settings with disparate health records and administrative infrastructures. Outside of tightly integrated delivery systems such as Kaiser-Permanente or geographically isolated settings where there is only one regional ED, patients in a single ambulatory care setting may seek care in multiple EDs, and EDs treat patients from many ambulatory practices. Gathering information on care transitions in these settings would require gaining access to all local record-keeping systems, which is logistically difficult if not impossible in many communities.

## Care coordination within EDs

Within the ED, providers often work in teams with physicians, nurses, and ED technicians. In these teams, information-sharing and division of tasks are the primary care coordination activity. Few studies have examined teamwork in EDs, but teamwork in the operating room (OR) has been studied extensively. Optimal communication among team members in the OR is usually appropriately timed, includes all necessary information, includes all relevant team members, and, by its conclusion, resolves the issue or question that triggered the communication.[7] Team members may not be able to judge the quality of their teamwork accurately; for example, a study of surgical staff found that surgeons rated the quality of their collaborations with OR nurses better than the nurses did.[8] Although simulation exercises are generally geared toward individual clinicians, teams can also engage in them together. Team-based simulation training can improve the quality of teamwork by increasing the frequency of positive behaviors such as maintaining a team structure and supporting team members with information.[9] Understanding teamwork in other hospital settings, like ORs, can shed light on how to optimize teamwork in the ED.

The composition of ED teams changes throughout the day as team members begin and end their shifts. Physicians, nurses, and others must share information, cooperate on tasks, and transfer information to their peers at change of shift. During this period, providers must quickly share essential information about a slate of patients that can orient oncoming providers to patients' clinical status, the process of their evaluation, and the plan for their eventual disposition. Providers conduct this process according to their training and personal preferences, which may involve handwritten notes, accessing an electronic health record, "walk rounds" where each patient is discussed at the bedside, or other strategies.[10] Physicians and nurses typically hand off care in separate meetings. A study of ED handoffs identified promising strategies for improving the quality of information-sharing during handoffs, including limiting interruptions, using "read-back" practices, including additional team members (not just the leaving and entering providers) in the handoff process, and encouraging providers to monitor their peers' handoffs. However, most of those strategies were never or rarely used.[11]

## Care coordination within hospitals

When patients in the ED require admission to the hospital, ED providers transfer care to an admitting provider. Sometimes this provider is the patient's continuity physician or specialist. However, increasingly, it is a hospital-based provider who may have no previous personal knowledge of the patient. In cases where the patient has not previously been hospitalized at that hospital, the ED record may be the sole, easily available source of objective information for the admitting provider.

This care transition is similar to ED shift change where one provider is transferring responsibility for a patient to another, but is complicated by several factors. The ED and admitting providers rarely speak face-to-face; these conversations are typically by telephone or may be asynchronous using a voicemail system.[12] It may be difficult to coordinate the timing of the information exchange optimally due to workflow differences between the ED and receiving physician. Smooth transfers of care between ED and inpatient providers may be impeded by cultural differences or differences in personal style and experiences, rather than guided by a standardized evidence-based approach.[13]

## Care coordination within communities

Care coordination with ambulatory (non-hospital-based) providers may involve patients being hospitalized under their care, or may involve the care of patients who are being discharged from the ED who require follow-up. Continuity providers often contribute information that may assist in better focusing their patient's ED care, and accept responsibility for coordinating the patient's ongoing care whether in the hospital or after discharge. It is estimated that ED providers face information gaps in nearly one-third of visits.[14] In one study, 87% of Australian ED physicians reported that a written management plan from a PCP had some influence on their ED patient management although telephone calls were preferable, and 89% reported that they usually or always responded to PCP's communications.[15,16] A British study reported that very few PCPs wanted detailed information on all ED visits, but almost 90% requested information about patients who would be following up with them for review or further treatment, and almost 80% requested a regular (weekly or monthly) list of all of their patients who had visited the ED.[17]

In a study of Canadian ED leaders, 85% reported that communication with community physicians needed at least some improvement.[18] UK general practitioners rated communication with their local ED 5.6 on a scale of 1–10,[19] and 19% of UK PCPs reported dissatisfaction with communication from their local ED while only 4% reported dissatisfaction with the quality of care provided.[20]

There is great variability among ED provider behavior in notifying community physicians about patients being treated in the ED and few objective guidelines for either party. ED providers most often use a telephone call for patients who are admitted or discharged with a need for immediate monitoring or follow-up, or a fax for patients whose post-discharge needs are more routine. Approaches that rely on patients transmitting information between physicians have been unsuccessful. A UK study showed that only around 60% of patients had delivered letters from the ED to their PCP within 2 weeks.[21] While ED physicians and PCPs who share an electronic health record often speak highly of its benefits, it does not guarantee seamless coordination of care.[22] Hospital-employed case managers have successfully assisted with care coordination for patients with frequent hospital admissions.

EDs have developed a variety of programs dedicated to coordinating care. A systematic review[23] identified 14 randomized controlled trials and 9 quasi-experimental studies describing care coordination interventions. Interventions included:
- Helping unassigned patients obtain a PCP;
- Helping patients schedule appointments with a new or existing PCP;
- Follow-up telephone calls to a patient after their discharge from the ED; and
- Transfer of detailed clinical information to PCPs about the ED visit.

These interventions were tested in a variety of clinical settings and showed variable effectiveness with no single approach being clearly dominant. Several studies showed a paradoxical increase in ED utilization for patients who received an ED-based care coordination intervention.

## Common problems with care coordination

Physicians are often not paid for care coordination that do not involve a face-to-face patient encounter. Conversing with another physician will contribute to the complexity of a visit and might merit a higher evaluation and management code (i.e., higher level of complexity resulting in a higher bill). However, such patients are likely to be high-complexity even if care coordination is not documented. Some PCPs' compensation models may reward care coordination that averts an inpatient admission, but ED providers do not have similar financial incentives at this time. Until recently, hospitals have had few incentives to support ED providers in care coordination efforts to avoid hospitalization, but as hospitals are now subject to financial penalties for high rates of readmission and in some cases participate in accountable care organizations, they may invest more in supporting ED-based care coordination in the future.

Care coordination can be disruptive to workflow for both ED and receiving providers. Coordination generally relies on synchronous communication between two providers who are each juggling competing demands. In practice, this means that a theoretically brief conversation to relay the details of a patient's clinical presentation and ensure timely follow-up may stretch over a much longer period, involving multiple interruptions as providers attempt to contact each other. Each interruption disrupts providers' workflow, adding to the possibility of error for both the patient whose care is being coordinated and also the providers' other patients. Alternative approaches to coordination rely on asynchronous communication, such as the use of emails and text messages, where providers can send and receive messages during breaks in between tasks.

Successful coordination may benefit from strong ongoing relationships between ED-based and community-based providers. Unfortunately, these relationships may be deteriorating. In a qualitative study,[24] both ED physicians and PCPs reported that rising hospitalist use had changed not just individual conversations around specific admissions, but also the ways they interact with community-based physicians in general. Community-based practitioners who previously cared for their own patients when they were admitted to the hospital reported they had regularly spent time at nearby hospitals, whether evaluating and writing orders on patients in the ED awaiting admission, or rounding on patients who are admitted on inpatient wards, attending grand rounds, or serving on committees. These interactions brought them into contact with ED providers on a regular basis, providing an opportunity for frequent informal interactions that built collegiality and trust. Over time, these community-based physicians reported, they visited the hospital less frequently after ceding primary responsibility for their admitted patients to dedicated hospitalists. For these physicians, and also for ED providers who reported observing similar changes in their community-based peers, the overall decline in interactions, rather than changes in the way specific discussions are conducted, has an adverse effect on care coordination.

For ED providers, fewer interactions with community-based providers may also add risk to care coordination. ED providers who do not have strong relationships with independent providers may be reluctant to trust unknown community providers to carry out complicated time-sensitive follow-up plans.

Other changes in ambulatory care practice shape care coordination in the ED. Most ambulatory physicians work in groups of three physicians or more; only one-third are in solo- or two-physician practices, and this proportion has fallen consistently for decades.[25] ED providers seeking to contact a patient's continuity provider may instead reach another member of that provider's practice, who may not have direct knowledge of the patient's clinical history or access to the patient's record. In many communities, several practices share call responsibilities, so the ED provider may be discussing a patient's care with a provider from an entirely different practice.[26] This may limit the utility of care coordination for ED providers, because they obtain less information when talking to a provider who does not know the patient.

## Conclusions

Care coordination is a necessary part of emergency care, but is underresourced and poorly studied. As the health care system evolves towards greater financial incentives for managing utilization and meeting quality standards, ED providers may be pressured to minimize errors, avoid admissions and readmissions, limit their use of some services, and shift others from the hospital to less costly settings. Emergency physicians will need to develop effective care coordination strategies that can help them ensure patients will have a safe discharge plan. Some of the barriers to care coordination (e.g., diminishing opportunities for regular interactions between ED-based and community-based providers) are part of larger trends in health care delivery and would be extremely difficult to reverse. ED providers may need to think creatively and develop new strategies for coordinating care.

# References

1 Schrag D, Xu F, Hanger M, Elkin E, Bickell N, Bach P. Fragmentation of care for frequently hospitalized urban residents. Med Care. 2006;44:560–7.

2 Haggerty JL, Reid RJ, Freeman GK, Starfield BH, Adair CF, McKendry R. Continuity of care: a multidisciplinary review. BMJ. 2003;327:1219–21. Cited in http://familymedicine.medschool.ucsf.edu/cepc/pdf/BodenheimerCareCoordination 2007.pdf (accessed 30 November 2013).

3 Saultz JW. Defining and measuring interpersonal continuity of care. Ann Fam Med. 2003;1:134–43.

4 National Quality Forum. NQF-Endorsed Definition and Framework for Measuring Care Coordination. Available at: http://216.122.138.39/pdf/reports/ambulatory_endorsed__definition.pdf. Cited in http://familymedicine.medschool.ucsf.edu/cepc/pdf/BodenheimerCareCoordination2007.pdf (accessed 30 November 2013).

5 Snow V, Beck D, Budnitz T, Miller DC, Potter J, Wears RL, et al. Transitions of care consensus policy statement American College of Physicians–Society of General Internal Medicine–Society of Hospital Medicine–American Geriatrics Society–American College of Emergency Physicians–Society of Academic Emergency Medicine. J Gen Intern Med. 2009;24:971–6.

6 Eligible Professional Meaning of Use Menu Set Measures. Available at: http://www.cms.gov/Regulations-and-Guidance/Legislation/EHRIncentivePrograms/downloads/8_Transition_of_Care_Summary.pdf (accessed 30 November 2013).

7 Lingard L, Espin S, Whyte S. Communication failures in the operating room: an observational classification of recurrent types and effects. Qual Saf Health Care. 2004;13:330–4.

8 Makary MA, Sexton JB, Freischlag JA, Holzmueller CG, Millman EA, Rowen L, et al. Operating room teamwork among physicians and nurses: teamwork in the eye of the beholder. J Am Coll Surg. 2006;202:746–52.

9 Shapiro MJ, Morey JC, Small SD, Langford V, Kaylor CJ, Jagminas L, et al. Simulation based teamwork training for emergency department staff: does it improve clinical team performance when added to an existing didactic teamwork curriculum? Qual Saf Health Care. 2004;13:417–21.

10 Laxmisan A, Hakimzada F, Sayan OR, Green RA, Zhang J, Patel VL. The multitasking clinician: decision-making and cognitive demand during and after team handoffs in emergency care. Int J Med Inform. 2007;76:801–11.

11 Behara R, Wears RL, Perry S, et al. A Conceptual Framework For Studying the Safety of Transitions in Emergency Care. Rockville, MD: Agency for Healthcare Research and Quality, 2005.

12 Horwitz LI, Meredith T, Schuur JD, Shah NR, Kulkarni RG, Jenq GY. Dropping the baton: a qualitative analysis of failures during the transition from emergency department to inpatient care. Ann Emerg Med. 2009;53:701–10.

13 Horwitz LI, Moin T, Green ML. Development and implementation of an oral sign-out curriculum for house staff. J Gen Intern Med. 2007;22:1470–4.

14 Stiell A, Fordter A, Stiell I, van Walraven C. Prevalence of information gaps in the emergency department and the effect on patient outcomes. Can Med Assoc J. 2003;169:1023–8.

15  Montalto M, Harris P, Rosengarten P. Survey of Australian emergency physicians' expectation of general practitioner referrals. Br J Gen Pract. 1993;43:277–80.

16  Crone P. Are preadmission general practitioner calls of value? A study in communication. N Z Med J. 1987;100:632–4.

17  Wass AR,Illingworth RN. What information do general practitioners want about accident and emergency patients? J Accid Emerg Med. 1996;13:406–8.

18  Stiell A, Forster A, Stiell I, van Walraven C. Maintaining continuity of care: a look at the quality of communication between Ontario emergency departments and community physicians. Can J Emerg Med. 2005;7:155–61.

19  Morrison WG, Pennybrook AG, Makower RM, Swann IJ. The general practitioner's use and expectations of an accident and emergency department. J R Soc Med. 1990;83:237–40.

20  Choyce MQ, Maitra AK. Satisfaction with the accident and emergency department: a postal survey of general practitioners' views. J Accid Emerg Med. 1996;13:280–2.

21  Sherry M, Edmunds S, Touquet R. The reliability of patients in delivering their letter from the hospital accident and emergency department to their general practitioner. Arch Emerg Med. 1985;2:161–4.

22  Lang E, Afilalo M, Vandal A, Boivin JF, Xue X, Colacone A, et al. Impact of an electronic link between the emergency department and family physicians: a randomized controlled trial. Can Med Assoc J. 2006;174:313–8.

23  Katz EB, Carrier ER, Umscheid CA, Pines JM. Comparative effectiveness of care coordination interventions in the emergency department: a systematic review. Ann Emerg Med. 2012;60:12–23.

24  Carrier E, Yee T, Holzwart RA. Coordination between emergency and primary care physicians. Center for Studying Health System Change, 2011.

25  HSC data Online-Physician Survey. Available at: http://hscdataonline.s-3.com/psurvey_r5.asp (accessed 30 November 2013).

26  O'Malley A, Samuel D, Bond A, Carrier E. After-hours care and its coordination with primary care in the US. J Gen Intern Med. 2012;27:1406–15.

# CHAPTER 12

# Payment reform in emergency care

## Janice Blanchard, Stephanie Donald, and Nathan Seth Trueger

Emergency Medicine and Health Policy, The George Washington University, USA

## Introduction

The United States' health care system is traditionally built on the fee-for-service (FFS) model where providers are reimbursed for individual elements of health care, such as each physician visit, diagnostic test, or procedure. Under the existing model of FFS health care, a single emergency department (ED) visit is typically billed and reimbursed as several individual components that comprise that visit. For example, a patient coming to the ED would have separately billed charges from the hospital (including nursing care), the emergency medicine physician, consulting physicians, and for any ancillary tests or procedures rendered. The fee system that reimburses facilities varies depending on whether an ED visit results in an admission or discharge. Providers are paid on a separate fee schedule based on diagnosis and intensity of services.[1,2]

This system of separate reimbursement for individual components of a visit does not always result in efficient, cost-effective, or high-quality care. FFS compensates providers for the volume of care, and can encourage the overuse of services. In the prevalent FFS model, payments are made regardless of the quality of the service delivered. Payment reform is designed to slow the rapidly growing costs of medical care largely associated with FFS medicine. Most payment reform initiatives were initially targeted towards the Medicare population, and later adopted by Medicaid and the private sector. In this chapter we discuss payment reform initiatives beginning with early models, followed by more recently proposed approaches. We also highlight the impact of payment reform on emergency

*Emergency Care and The Public's Health*, First Edition.
Edited by Jesse M. Pines, Jameel Abualenain, James Scott and Robert Shesser.
© 2014 John Wiley & Sons, Ltd. Published 2014 by John Wiley & Sons, Ltd.

medicine as well as overall challenges to the implementation of various measures.

## Early payment reform initiatives

The earliest payment reform initiatives focused on limiting costs with less emphasis on ensuring quality. Many of these reform initiatives had a number of shortcomings from the perspective of both the provider and patient: the prospective payment system, capitation models, and relative value scales.

### Prospective payment system

One of the earliest reforms was the prospective payment system, initially established in 1983, which reimburses hospitals a fixed payment for a hospital admission rather than individually billed services that occur during an admission.[3] For a given diagnosis, costs are determined prospectively based on prior average costs for the usual resources and length of stay associated with a particular diagnosis. The expected services and resources associated with a given diagnosis are grouped into Diagnosis Related Groups (DRGs). The DRG system prospectively determines costs associated with a diagnosis, with the index DRG for comparison being the cost of the average Medicare beneficiary nationwide. The DRG is adjusted based on a number of factors, including severity of illness, regional market level factors (such as higher wages of hospital staff), as well as other hospital characteristics (including whether a hospital is a teaching hospital, is in a rural area, or serves a disproportionately higher number of low income patients).[3]

This system as originally introduced was not effective in reducing costs because of adverse incentives. Specifically, because DRGs payments are bundled based on an episode of care, hospitals obtain a profit margin when admitted patients have a shorter stay and use fewer services than predicted by the DRG for that particular diagnosis. Hospitals were therefore more likely to code patients for DRGs associated with a higher severity of illness in order to still benefit from a favorable margin. Patients admitted from EDs tend to be sicker and their cases more complicated than patients admitted electively with the same DRG diagnosis; therefore ED admissions in general offer a somewhat lower profit margin than elective admissions.[4-7] Also, because physician services were not included in the DRG system, provider billing did not decrease. As a result, although length of stay did decrease for Medicare patients after DRGs were rolled out, there was no decrease in overall costs.[1] Within the first years after introduction of the DRG system, hospital Medicare spending exceeded $400 million per year more than originally projected.

## Capitation models

Capitation allows a set predetermined payment to be paid for each patient member during a specific time period. An early capitation model commonly associated with managed care plans was first introduced in the 1980s.[8] Capitation models are designed to contain costs by reducing excess services by establishing a set payment per patient or, in the case of managed care plans, per member per month. Providers have the incentive to reduce ED visits and provider referrals, when such services are included in the capitated payment.[9]

Early models of capitation, however, did not appropriately risk adjust for patients based on severity of illness; this created adverse incentives where providers were more likely to select healthier patients to participate in their practice panels to help control costs.[10] Early capitation models limited the ability of patients to visit the ED for care by requiring preauthorization before a visit or denial of ED claims considered inappropriate by managed care organizations.[11] The prudent layperson standard, passed as part of the Patient Access to Responsible Care Act of 1997, helped address limitations on ED reimbursement by allowing patients to receive emergency care without preauthorization as considered necessary for medical stabilization (based on what a "prudent layperson" considered was emergent).[12] Capitation also resulted in a negative reaction among consumers to the limitation of choice associated with closed panel managed care plans as a mechanism of reducing costs.[13]

## Relative value scales

While DRGs are aimed at curtailing spending for hospital-based services, relative value scales target excessive growth in costs of physician services. Congress passed the Omnibus Budget Reconciliation Act of 1989, which mandated use of relative value scales in reforming physician payment under Medicare; such resource-based relative value scales (RBRVS), were also later adopted by private insurers. RBRVS are weights based on the resources required to provide a given procedure, including time, geographic variability, and malpractice expenses.[14] Congress adopted a conversion factor multiplied by the relative value unit of a procedure to determine final payment to providers. This conversion factor is designed to limit the growth in overall Medicare spending and was intended to be updated annually based on the Medicare sustainable growth rate (SGR).[15] The SGR is a formula linked to growth in the annual gross domestic product (GDP) and was adopted in 1997. It followed an earlier formula to cut costs, called the Value Performance Standards.[16]

The problem with the RBRVS is that this scale incorporates effort (i.e., level of complicity and time involved to complete a procedure) without accounting for quality or appropriateness of a procedure. In addition, there has been a delay in implementation to the SGR in order to avoid large cuts in Medicare physician fees as growth in healthcare costs have significantly outpaced GDP. Because Medicare fee schedules are adjusted annually, Congress has to vote each year on whether the SGR should be implemented.[17] It has voted against implantation each year since 2003; the cost savings measures proposed by the SGR have therefore not been adopted, suggesting a need for repeal or redesign.

## Newer payment reform models

Newer approaches to payment reform seek to introduce quality while achieving cost savings. These include care delivery systems that coordinate care to achieve high-quality lower cost care some with shared savings to the provider, such as Accountable Care Organizations (ACO) and Patient Centered Medical Homes (PCMH). Other approaches include models to adjust the mechanism and incentives associated with physician payments, such as bundled payments and pay for performance measures. Many of the newer payment reform models are evolutions of previous approaches, offering a hybrid of elements present in prior initiatives.[18] For example, the PCMH was an idea introduced as early as 1967 by the American Academy of Pediatrics to coordinate care for children with special health needs.[19]

### Care delivery systems
#### Accountable care organizations
The Affordable Care Act of 2010 set forth guidelines for the Centers for Medicare and Medicaid Services (CMS) to develop and implement ACOs.[20] ACOs are defined as integrated health care delivery systems comprised of providers and systems (such as acute care hospitals, primary care providers, specialists, etc.) that voluntarily join together to provide coordinated care to at least 5000 patients who receive Original Fee-for-Service Medicare. Currently, there are three categories of ACOs operating under Medicare: the Medicare Shared Savings Program, the Advance Payment Model, and the Pioneer ACO Model. Central to each of these types of ACOs are the concepts of improving health outcomes and saving money, by providing high-quality seamless care at a lower cost.[21]

The Medicare Shared Savings Program is the original program designed to encourage healthcare providers and acute care hospitals to join together to create an ACO. The basic premise is that an ACO that meets targeted quality measures and provides care at a cost lower than a CMS estimate will share the achieved savings with CMS. Each ACO must assume either a one-sided shared savings or a two-sided shared savings, based upon how much financial risk the ACO wants to take. If an ACO assumes a two-sided shared savings model, providers are eligible to receive a higher percentage of the savings they achieve through providing lower cost care than if they assumed a one-sided model. However, under the two-sided shared savings model, if an ACO incurs financial losses to Medicare, it will also be responsible for repaying a proportion of those losses to CMS, while under the one-sided model, providers would not be responsible for repaying losses.[22]

The Advance Payment Model is a subset of the Shared Savings Program that provides financial support to smaller, physician-owned, and rural practices to form ACOs. These smaller, generally lower funded organizations require more financial support to create the infrastructure needed to run an ACO, such as increased staffing, electronic health records, and administrative services; thus, they are granted their presumed share of savings in advance, so that they may use the funding to create an infrastructure capable of delivering seamless care (i.e., coordination of care that facilitates a smooth transition of a patient from the hospital to the home at discharge, insuring continuity of care to the outpatient setting).[23,24]

The Pioneer ACO Model consists of 32 select ACOs around the United States that already provide high-quality coordinated care. These health care systems were chosen to serve as innovative leaders in the seamless care movement. Through the Pioneer ACO Model, CMS and the Centers for Medicare and Medicaid Innovation (CMMI) are piloting reimbursement structures based upon a benchmark expenditure level derived from the historical health care expenditures of prospectively aligned Medicare beneficiaries in a traditional FFS payment system. In 2011–2013, CMS will assess their cost-effectiveness, ability to deliver coordinated care, and patients' health outcomes.[25]

Only if an ACO achieves savings and meets quality performance metrics will it qualify to receive a proportion of the savings. There are 33 quality measures that an ACO must meet in order to share in savings achieved over the course of 1 year. These quality measures are grouped into four nationally recognized categories:

1 Patient/caregiver experience;
2 Care coordination and patient safety;
3 Preventive health; and
4 At-risk populations.

In an attempt to assist newly formed ACOs with adjusting to working together to achieve savings and meet quality measures, in year 1 of existence, the ACO is rewarded on a pay-for-reporting basis. In years 2 and 3, a graduated responsibility for meeting the quality measures is set forth, with year 2 requiring pay-for-reporting (P4R) for eight of the quality measures and pay-for-performance (P4P, discussed later in the chapter in more detail) on 25 of the measures, and year 3 P4P on 32 quality measures, and P4R on one measure. Every year, a risk-adjusted benchmark for meeting quality measures will be set by CMS, and an ACO will be responsible for meeting this goal in order to receive its proportion of shared savings from Medicare.[26]

### Patient-centered medical home

PCMH is a model of primary care delivery led by a central primary care provider (PCP), designed to deliver coordinated care across various healthcare settings. The PCMH model is similar to ACOs; its goals are summarized by the "Triple Aim": to improve the experience of care, improve the health of populations, and reduce per capita costs of healthcare.[27] The American College of Physicians, the American Academy of Pediatrics, the American Academy of Family Physicians, and the American Osteopathic Association developed seven joint principles to describe the PCMH:

1 A personal physician;
2 Physician-directed medical practice;
3 Whole-person orientation;
4 Coordination and integration of care;
5 Attention to quality and safety;
6 Enhanced access to care; and
7 Payment that appropriately recognizes the value added to patients who have a PCMH.[28]

The goal of the PCMH is to improve primary care by providing each patient with one PCP who will coordinate all care that a patient needs, while meeting national quality benchmarks set forth by CMS.

The PCMH model is based on support and adequate resources within the primary care setting. When providing high-quality seamless care, the PCP must ensure that communication between all providers is facilitated and that patients are able to access the healthcare system for all of their needs in a way that does not result in fragmented care. It has been recognized that much of the time a PCP spends coordinating care is outside of the patient visit, and thus it goes uncompensated, but in the PCMH model, payment reform that incentivizes the core aspects of care coordination is key to ensuring that PCPs and other support staff who assist with coordinating care are compensated for this time.

Early evidence from the CMS's Medicare Physician Group Practice Demonstration (PGDP) suggest promising results in cost savings and improved quality.[29] Innovators in the PCMH movement, such as the

Geisinger Health System, Intermountain Healthcare Medical Group, and Community Care of North Carolina have all shown data in support of potential success of the seamless care model. For example, Geisinger estimated a $3.7 million net savings, Intermountain demonstrated a 10% reduction in total hospitalizations, and Community Care of North Carolina achieved a 40% reduction in asthma admissions, all through PCMH models of care.[30] A study of 10 physician groups that initially participated in the PGDP showed a significant reduction in savings from acute care admissions. Although data from the 10 hospitals combined showed no significant change in ED visits, there was a reduction in the 30-day readmission rate, with the effect most marked for Medicare–Medicaid dual eligible enrollees. Individual sites that produced the biggest impact on savings, however, did see reductions in ED visits.[31]

Although there have been favorable early results of the Medicare PGDP, in general more evidence is needed to evaluate the effectiveness of the PCMH model across diverse patient settings. Many early PCMH models did not include sufficient evaluation components to assess effectiveness adequately; of those that did, most only followed patients for relatively short time periods (less than 3 years).[32] The Agency for Healthcare Research and Quality and Mathematica Policy Research recently completed an evaluation of early models that had addressed three of five core principles of the PCMH (patient-centered, comprehensive, coordinated, accessible and continuous improvement through a systems-based approach to quality and safety) and that also included a quantitative evaluation of a Triple Aim outcome. Of 14 studies of 12 early PCMH interventions, the evaluation found mixed resulted in terms of costs and utilization. Most of the positive effects were only seen among high needs patients. Hospitalizations decreased in three of the studies for high needs patients but there were no significant decreases in ED utilization, except in one study with a high needs Medicare population. Costs were also found to decrease only among a high needs population in the first year. Among patients with lower medical needs, costs were found to either increase or had inconclusive changes.[32,33] More rigorous studies are needed to fully evaluate the impact of the PCMH in the future, including studies that have sufficient sample sizes to examine the effect in patient subgroups and that follow patients over a longer study period.[32,33]

## Physician payment initiatives
### Bundled payments

Unlike the traditional FFS model in which payment is made for services separately (such as procedure, diagnostic test, physician services), payments can be grouped or "bundled" together. There are a variety of models for bundling payments, but they share the same concept: providers are paid a single lump-sum for all care for a defined episode or period of time. Therefore, providers take on the financial risk and are encouraged to provide efficient high-quality care, as unexpected costs to treat complications are not further compensated.

The major drawback with bundled payments is that the incentives are aligned for providers to deliver as little care as they can. While this should bring down overall costs, providers may be reluctant to provide care when needed. Further, as noted in the discussion of capitation models, as providers carry the majority of the financial risk, they may select healthier patients who are less likely to require more care and exceed the bundled payment. To ensure appropriate care is delivered when needed, bundled payment systems are often implemented in conjunction with pay-for-performance systems to serve as a safety benchmark.

Bundled payments are not the same as coordinated care (PCMH and ACO). Whereas coordinated care systems "bundle" the delivery of care under a network of providers, payments may still be structured as FFS. If the overall costs are lower than projected, then providers keep a portion of the savings. On the other hand, bundled payments refer to a single payment for all of the care provided during an episode of care or period of time. If the cost of providing care during that episode is lower than the payment, then the providers keep the difference. Bundled payments inherently encourage care coordination, as a sizable portion of health care involves multiple providers who participate in an episode of care and therefore share in the bundled payment; coordination is therefore encouraged in order to provide efficient care at the lowest cost. Currently, most physician payments are FFS, but Medicare (and many private insurers) has been paying hospitals for each inpatient admission with prospective bundled payments under the DRG system since the early 1980s.[34]

### Episode bundles

Payments can be bundled for a single surgical procedure or episode of illness. For example, a bundled payment for an acute myocardial infarction would cover the hospital admission, testing including ECG, labs and imaging, treatment including catheterization and stent placement, medications, and post-discharge follow-up, including treatment of complications and an entire readmission if necessary. One example by Medicare defines an episode of care as beginning 3 days prior to hospitalization, extending to 30 days post-discharge.[35] This differs from the DRG system in that the lump payment is comprehensive, including physician and hospital fees. As each element of care is not individually reimbursed, providers are incentivized to order only necessary tests and treatments, shorten lengths of stay, and minimize complications. In 2006, Geisinger Health Systems successfully implemented ProvenCare, a bundled payment system for cardiac surgery, which modestly decreased complications, length of stay and readmissions, while bringing down costs.[36]

Alternatively, bundled payments can also be capitated, paying a set amount for each patient over a period of time, either a single lump sum for each patient, or for the care of a patient's chronic disease over a period of time, such as for an individual's diabetes care for the year. Programs such as the Patient Choice System have demonstrated small decreases in premiums and overall costs while maintaining quality in a number of health care markets.[35] The Affordable Care Act introduced episode-based bundles for some surgical procedures under Medicare. The CMMI has awarded grants to pilot a number of demonstration projects for various capitated chronic condition and global payment models.[37]

### Pay for performance and value-based purchasing

Another approach to improve the FFS system is to tie payments to the quality of care that physicians and hospitals provide, or "pay for performance" (P4P). Whereas CMS uses the term "value-based purchasing" to refer to an overall philosophy of improving quality while containing cost growth, thereby improving value, P4P refers specifically to tying payments to quality measures. Quality measures can be tied to process measures (such as the now-defunct time to first antibiotic dose for ED patients with pneumonia) or to outcomes, usually risk-adjusted mortality. While outcome-based measures are theoretically preferred, current risk-adjustment models for estimating a hospital's expected mortality perform inconsistently at best.[38] Process-based measures currently predominate, largely because they are simpler to measure; however, they show only a small window on clinical performance, allowing providers to focus efforts on meeting quality measures without necessarily improving care or patient outcomes, effectively gaming the system.[39]

Currently, most P4P measures are developed by medical specialty organizations: the American Medical Association's Physician Consortium for Performance Improvement (PCPI) which includes 97 member specialty organizations (including the American College of Emergency Physicians); the independent National Committee for Quality Assurance, which now collaborates with PCPI; the Ambulatory Care Quality Alliance, which includes the American Academy of Family Physicians and the American College of Physicians as members; and, the National Quality Forum (NQF), whose role includes analyzing measures developed by other groups.[40,41] Insurers then decide whether to base payments on these measures; notably, CMS adopts many of the NQF-supported measures, and private insurers often follow suit.[41]

CMS is implementing P4P in a number of ways. First, the Hospital Value Based Purchasing (HVBP) will adjust a hospital's Medicare payments by as much as 1% in fiscal year 2014 (up to 2% in 2017 when fully phased in) based on a number of process-based quality measures in the preceding year. Measures relevant to the ED include meeting a 90-minute door to balloon time for acute myocardial infarction.[42] CMS has demonstrated responsiveness to ED provider feedback about its quality measures, particularly those that are thought to negatively impact everyday practice. For example, CMS withdrew the time-to-antibiotic for pneumonia measure, postponed implementation of a metric of ED rates of CT scans for atraumatic headache for further refinement, and incorporated measures to improve ED crowding.[43]

The HVBP score will be combined with hospital's performance on the Hospital Consumer Assessment of Healthcare Providers and Systems Survey (HCAHPS) patient satisfaction survey to determine the payment adjuster.[18,40] Linking payments to patient satisfaction surveys has drawn criticism, as patients' subjective experience may not be related to the quality of clinical care, as well as inconsistency due to response bias and small sample sizes.[44]

Similarly, CMS's Hospital Readmissions Reduction Program aims to decrease readmissions to the hospital within 30-days of hospital discharge. Under the program, hospitals will lose up to 3% of their total Medicare reimbursement (phased in from 2013 to 2016) if they exceed risk-adjusted target 30-day readmission rates for pneumonia, heart failure, and acute myocardial infarction, with CMS expanding the list of target diagnoses over time.[45] While only patients with the initial targeted diagnoses are affected, the measure includes readmissions for any reason. Additionally, critical access hospitals are least well equipped to prevent readmissions, putting vulnerable populations at risk.[46,47]

## Emergency medicine and payment reform

While the Readmissions Reduction Program and HVBP may only have a small impact on individual hospitals,[47] more than 2000 hospitals are facing reduced Medicare payments in the first year alone.[48] Emergency physicians will likely face pressure to avoid admitting recently discharged patients, despite having little control over the factors that necessitate readmission.[49] Although a great deal of focus has been on reducing hospital readmissions within 30 days, a significant number of discharged patients will have an ED visit related to their index hospitalization during this same time period. In many cases these ED visits result in treatment and subsequent discharge.[50] Given this high rate of ED use post discharge, there may be more pressure for ED providers to place patients on observation units or to offer stabilization within the ED to avoid readmission. Care coordination prior to discharge, particularly for vulnerable populations at highest risk for revisits (such as persons with mental illness and substance abuse disorders) will be important to reduce the risk of recurrent ED use and associated readmissions.[50]

Additionally, emergency medical care may not fit easily into a bundled payment system. Even for well-defined episodes of care, patients often seek care at multiple hospitals.[51] Similarly, disease-specific capitation may be confounded by overlapping interrelated conditions (e.g., is an acute myocardial infarction included in the annual bundle for diabetes care?).[52] Further, EDs may be pressured to disposition patients based not just on their clinical symptoms, but on how a visit fits into an episode: if admission would trigger a new episode and payment, then the incentives are equivalent to the current volume-based FFS system, but if it would be included in a current episode whose bundle has already been triggered, no further reimbursements would be received.[49] While bundled payments, coordinated care, and P4P seek to align incentives to minimize complications and overuse while improving quality, most EDs are uniquely constrained by the Emergency Treatment and Active Labor Act and are unable to select patients or influence care-seeking behavior for the most part.[52] As bundled payments are distributed to care networks and hospitals, institutions will be responsible for distributing payments among providers, and hospitals tend to overestimate the costs of ED care while underestimating rates of patient insurance and revenue generated from EDs.[53] Given that ED care is typically viewed as high cost episodic care and may not be considered a central part of the outpatient care coordination model, some EDs may be in danger of being marginalized in negotiating a role in the ACO model.[54]

## Challenges

### Information exchange

In order to ensure that payment reform systems are effective and help encourage coordination of care, adequate record sharing is needed, ideally electronically. Most notably, these systems must operate with an electronic health record (EHR) system, in order to provide seamless and complete access to patient information for every provider caring for a patient within the group. Health information technology lies at the core of low-cost high-quality seamless healthcare. This is particularly true in the ED setting, where an existing relationship with a patient may not exist. Access to EHR in the ED can potentially reduce redundant medical services, subsequent length of stay and avoidable readmissions.[54,55] An EHR system traditionally costs in the order of millions of dollars alone, but there is some evidence that it may help to reduce medication errors, improve health screening, and enhance communication among many health care providers.[56] However, EHRs are still relatively new and will require further study, particularly in the ED setting where care priorities often differ from inpatient settings, for which some EHR platforms are designed. In an effort to encourage the adoption of EHRs, hospitals are eligible for federal incentive payments if they demonstrate meaningful use of the EHR. Hospitals must attest to implementing EHR across a range of measures, many of which are relevant to emergency medicine including computerized physician order entry, patient-specific problem lists, and capability to send surveillance data to relevant public health agencies. Hospitals must also report on various quality metrics, such as ED length of stay, to qualify.[57] In turn, EHRs may help improve future collection of metrics to help better track quality in the long term.

## Assumption of risk

It will also be important in shared payment systems to coordinate incentives across hospitals as well as different categories of providers. Bundled payments require shared risk and distribution of savings across multiple entities such as hospitals, provider groups, and individual providers. Determining provider collaboration and distribution of financial risk as well as payments is a challenge that requires advance planning and forethought by participating entities and institutions.[10,58] As many acute episodes of care occur across multiple provider settings, it may be difficult to assess the level of involvement and risk assigned to the ED.[58]

## Evidence-based care

One of the biggest challenges to initiating payment reform initiatives will be ensuring that care is evidence-based. In particular, although care may meet the quality and cost goals associated with new payment reform measures, it will be important to make sure care improves healthcare outcomes. It will also be important to ensure that providers are aware of evidence-based approaches to care that improve outcomes and to ensure that provider knowledge is reconciled with patient expectations.[59] In the ED, this may involve the use of clinical decision rules may help reduce care – such as diagnostic testing – that may otherwise be safely avoided.[60]

## Regional variations in care

Critics have expressed concerns that regional spending patterns vary greatly, but that the ACO payment model is based on national Medicare spending patterns. Proponents of this method maintain that areas of higher spending, beyond that of the national average, will be forced to contain their costs, whereas areas of lower spending than the national average are projected to enjoy greater cost savings.[61] EDs in geographic areas with higher than average spending may be under greater pressure to reduce readmissions and to increase cost savings even with of a sicker patient population. However, the concern stems from the fact that an ACO with higher spending may incur significant losses greater than projected, despite efforts to improve quality, because they operate within a market with higher average spending rates. This issue is heavily debated, and data from the Pioneer ACO project will answer many questions surrounding spending and cost savings. If the projection is in fact truth, the potential economic losses (translated to risk), may discourage ACO expansion in areas of higher-than-average spending.

## Vulnerable and high-risk populations

Finally, the ACO concept has the potential to worsen health disparities and access to care for vulnerable patient populations. As every ACO must care for at least 5000 patients, and these patients are all different medically – some have chronic illnesses, some are disabled, some are very poor, others are wealthy, and some are healthy and only see their primary care provider once per year or less for a health maintenance examination. By agreeing to care for a patient, the ACO inherently assumes that it can provide care for a patient that meets CMS's standards for cost and quality, after a risk adjustment for a sicker patient population.[36] If an ACO fails to meet the quality and cost standards (e.g., through missed quality measures, hospital readmissions, multiple ED visits or other high-cost health care expenditures), then it will not enjoy the proposed cost savings, and could potentially incur financial losses depending the ACO category. Thus, there is potential for ACOs to avoid caring for high-risk patient populations, further increase health care disparities, and decrease access to healthcare for vulnerable patient populations.[62]

## Conclusions

Though payment reform measures have the potential to cut costs and improve quality for many Americans, a tremendous investment is needed in order to create a seamless care delivery system, and financial risks lie at the structural, informational, and care delivery levels. Providers must invest in the infrastructure needed to provide seamless care. Time and expertise both in health care management and health care delivery are needed, as well as bricks and mortar to house the facilities needed to provide patient care.

Overall, seamless healthcare delivery models promise innovative new methods for improving health outcomes and reducing health care spending. Providers and health care systems willing to make the investments required to expand these models of care delivery may lead the national effort to streamline how care is provided care in the United States.

## References

1 Rhinehardt UE. How do hospitals get paid? A primer. New York Times, 2009. Available at: http://economix.blogs.nytimes.com/2009/01/23/how-do-hospitals-get-paid-a-primer/ (accessed 30 November 2013).

2 Scarrow AM. Physician reimbursement under Medicare. Medscape. 2002. Available at: http://www.medscape.com/viewarticle/433293_2 (accessed 30 November 2013).

3 Altman S. The lessons of medicare's prospective payment system show that the bundled payment program faces challenges. Health Aff. 2012;31:1923–30.

4 McHugh M, Regenstein M, Siegel B. The profitability of medicare admissions based on source of admission. Acad Emerg Med. 2008;15:900–7.

5 Schneider SM, Asplin BR. Form follows finance: emergency department admissions and hospital operating margins. Acad Emerg Med. 2008;15:959–60.

6 Munoz E, Mulloy K, Goldstein J, Josephson J, Tenenbaum N, Wise L. Physicians' patient load per DRG, the consumption of hospital resources, and the incentives of the DRG prospective payment system. Acad Med. 1990;65:533–8.

7 Prospective Payment Assessment Commission. 1985. Internal report. ProPAC.

8 Glied S. Managed care: NBER Working Paper 7205. National Bureau of Economic Research, 1999. Available at: http://www.nber.org/papers/w7205 (accessed 30 November 2013).

9 Zuvekas SH, Hill SC. Does capitation matter? Impacts on access, use, and quality. Inquiry. 2004;41:316–35.

10 Miller HD. From volume to value: better ways to pay for health care. Health Aff. 2009;28:1418–28.

11 Gresenz CR, Studdert DM. Disputes over coverage of emergency department services: a study of two health maintenance organizations. Ann Emerg Med. 2004;43:155–62.

12 Asplin B. Controversial company: the prudent layperson standard and the patients' bill of rights. Ann Emerg Med. 2000;35:304–7.

13 Mechanic RE, Altman SH, McDonogh JE. The new era of payment reform spending targets, and cost containment in Massachusetts: early lessons for the nation. Health Aff. 2012;31:2334–42.

14 Dove HG. Use of the resource-based relative value scale for private insurers. Health Aff. 1994;13:193–201.

15  American Academy of Pediatrics Committee on Coding and Nomenclature. Application of the resource-based relative value scale system to pediatrics. Pediatrics. 2008;122:1395–400.

16  Ginsberg PB. Provider payment incentives and delivery system reform. In: The Health Care Delivery System: A Blueprint for Reform. Center for American Progress and Institute on Medicine as a Profession, 2008.

17  Laugesen MJ. Siren song: physicians, congress and Medicare fees. J Health Polit Policy Law 2009;34:157–79.

18  Rosenthal M. Beyond pay for performance: emerging models. N Engl J Med 2008;359:1197–200.

19  Inglehart JK. No place like home: testing a new model of care delivery. N Engl J Med 2008;359:1200–2.

20  Patient Protection and Affordable Care Act of 2010. Pub. L. No. 111-148, §3022 124.

21  Department of Health and Human Services. Accountable Care Organizations: Improving Care Coordination for People with Medicare. Available at: http://www.healthcare.gov/news/factsheets/2011/03/accountablecare03312011a.html (accessed 30 November 2012).

22  American Hospital Association. 2010 committee on research. AHA research synthesis report: Accountable Care Organization. Chicago: American Hospital Association, 2010.

23  Centers for Medicare and Medicaid Innovation. Advanced Payment ACO Model. Available at: http://innovations.cms.gov/initiatives/ACO/Advance-Payment/index.html (accessed 6 Jan 2013).

24  Spehar, A.M., Campbell R.R.,Cherrie C. et al. (2013) Seamless care: safe transitions from hospital to home. www.ahrq.gov/downloads/pub/advances/vol1/spehar.pdf (accessed 12 June 2013).

25  Centers for Medicare and Medicaid Innovation. (2012) Pioneer Accountable Care Organization Model: General Fact Sheet. Available at: http://innovations.cms.gov/initiatives/ACO/index.html (accessed 30 November 2013).

26  RTI International and Telligen. Accountable Care Organization 2012 Program Analysis: Quality Performance Standards Narrative Measure Specifications, Final Report. 2011. RTI Project Number 0213195.000.004.

27  Patient Centered Primary Care Collaborative. Achieving the Triple Aim: Quality, Outcomes and Cost. Available at: http://www.pcpcc.net/guide/evidence-quality (accessed 30 November 2013).

28  American Academy of Family Physicians, American Academy of Pediatrics, American College of Physicians, American Osteopathic Association. Joint Principles of the Patient-Centered Medical Home. 2007. Available at: http://www.acponline.org/running_practice/delivery_and_payment_models/pcmh/demonstrations/jointprinc_05_17.pdf (accessed 30 November 2013).

29  Centers for Medicare and Medicaid Services. Physician Group Practice Demonstration: Physician Groups Continue to Improve Quality and Generate Savings Under Medicare Pay-for-Performance Demonstration. Baltimore: Department of Health and Human Services, 2011: pp. 1–9.

30  Grumbach K, Brodenheimer T, Grundy P. Outcomes of implementing patient centered medical home interventions: a review of the evidence from prospective evaluation studies in the United States. Patient-Centered Primary Care

Collaborative. 2010. Available at: http://www.pcpcc.net/files/pcmh_evidence_outcomes_2009.pdf (accessed 6 January 2013).

31 Colla CH. Spending differences associated with the Medicare physician group practice demonstration. J Am Med Assoc. 2012;308:1015–23.

32 Peikes D, Zutshi A, Dale S, Lundquist E. The medical home: what we know, what do we need to know? A review of the evidence. Mathematica Policy Research Webinar, 2012. Available at: http://www.ehcca.com/presentations/MedHome20120124/peikes-zutshi.pdf (accessed 30 November 2013).

33 Peikes D, Zutshi A, Genevro J, Smith K, Parchman M, Meyers D. Early evidence on the patient centered medical home. Mathematica Policy Research for the Agency for Healthcare Research and Quality, 2012. Available at: http://pcmh.ahrq.gov/portal/server.pt/community/pcmh__home/1483/pcmh_evidence___evaluation_v2 (accessed 30 November 2013).

34 Frakt AB, Mayes R. Beyond capitation: how new payment experiments seek to find the "sweet spot" in amount of risk providers and payers bear. Health Aff. 2012;31:1951–8.

35 Kaiser Family Foundation. Focus on Health Reform: Summary of New Health Reform Law. Available at: www.kff.org/healthreform/upload/8061.pdf (accessed 30 November 2013).

36 Mechanic RE, Altman SH. Payment reform options: episode payment is a good place to start. Health Aff. 2009;28:262–71.

37 Korda H, Eldridge GN. Payment incentives and integrated care delivery: levers for health system reform and cost containment. Inquiry. 2011;48:277–87.

38 Pronovost PJ, Lilford R. Analysis and commentary: a road map for improving the performance of performance measures. Health Aff. 2011;30:569–73.

39 Conn J. US News & World retort: JCAHO study questions magazine's ranking system. Mod Healthc 2006;36:10.

40 Ferris TG, Vogeli C, Marder J, Sennett CS, Campbell EG. Physician specialty societies and the development of physician performance measures. Health Aff. 2007;26:1712–9.

41 Dorrity M. New Methods of Payment. In: Schlicher NR (ed.) Emergency Medicine Advocacy Handbook, 2nd edn. Irving, TX: Emergency Medicine Residents' Association, 2011: p. 49.

42 MS Quality Initiatives Patient Assessment Instruments. Frequently Asked Questions: Hospital Value-Based Purchasing Program. Available at: http://www.cms.gov/Medicare/Quality-Initiatives-Patient-Assessment-Instruments/hospital-value-based-purchasing/downloads/HVBPFAQ022812.pdf (accessed 30 November 2013).

43 Requirements for Reporting of Hospital OQR Data for the CY 2014 Payment Determination and Subsequent Years. Vol 77 Federal Register. 2012;221:68481–3.

44 Fenton JJ, Jerant AF, Bertakis KD, Franks P. The cost of satisfaction: a national study of patient satisfaction, health care utilization, expenditures, and mortality. Arch Int Med. 2012;172:405–11.

45 Berenson RA, Paulus RA, Kalman NS. Medicare's readmissions-reduction program: a positive alternative. N Engl J Med 2012;366:1364–6.

46 Joynt KE, Rosenthal MB. Hospital value-based purchasing: will Medicare's new policy exacerbate disparities? Circ 2012;5:148–9.

47 Atkinson JG. Flaws in the Medicare readmission penalty. N Engl J Med 2012;367:2056–7.

48 Fiegl C. 2,200 hospitals face Medicare pay penalty for readmissions. Am Med News. 2012. Available at: http://www.amaassn.org/amednews/2012/08/27/gvsb0827.htm (accessed 30 November 2013).

49 Asplin BR. Value-based purchasing and hospital admissions: doing the right thing isn't easy. Ann Emerg Med. 2010;56:258–60.

50 Vashi AA, Fox JP, Carr BG, D'Onofrio G, Pines JM, Ross JS, et al. Use of hospital-based acute care among patients recently discharged from the hospital. J Am Med Assoc. 2013;309:364–71.

51 de Brantes F, D'Andrea G, Rosenthal MB. Should health care come with a warranty? Health Aff. 2009;28:678–87.

52 Wiler JL, Beck D, Asplin BR, Granovsky M, Moorhead J, Pilgrim R, et al. Episodes of care: is emergency medicine ready? Ann Emerg Med. 2012;59:351–7.

53 Rabin E, Kocher K, McClelland M, Pines J, Hwang U, Rathlev N, et al. Solutions to emergency department 'boarding' and crowding are underused and may need to be legislated. Health Aff. 2012;31:1757–66.

54 Daniel GW, Ewen E, Wiley VJ, Reese CL, Shirazi F, Malone DC. Efficiency and economic benefits of a payer-based electronic health record in an emergency department. Acad Emerg Med. 2010;17:824–33.

55 Ofir BA, Itamar A, Moshe L. The impact of EHR and HIE on reducing avoidable admissions: controlling main differential diagnoses. BMC Med Inform Decis Mak 2013;13:49.

56 Fleming NS, Culler SD, McCorkle R, Becker ER, Ballard DJ. The financial and non-financial costs of implementing electronic health records in primary care practices. Health Aff. 2011;30:481–9.

57 Genes NG. The wired department: M.U. and you. Emerg Phys Mon. 2010. Available at: http://www.epmonthly.com/archives/features/mu-and-you/ (accessed 30 November 2013).

58 Komisar HL, Feder J, Ginsburg PB. "Bundling" payment for episodes of hospital care: Issues and recommendations for the new pilot program in Medicare. Center for American Progress, 2011. Available at: http://www.americanprogress.org/wp-content/uploads/issues/2011/07/pdf/medicare_bundling.pdf (accessed 30 November 2013).

59 AMA Innovators Committee. Early innovators share what they have learned. American Medical Association, 2012. Available at: http://www.hcms.org/uploadedFiles/Business_of_Medicine/ACO/AMA%20delivery-reform-white-paper-May2012.pdf (accessed 30 November 2013).

60 Agrawal P, Koaowsky JM. Pooja clinical practice guidelines in the emergency department. Emerg Med Clin North Am. 2009;27:555–67.

61 McWilliams JM, Song Z. Implications for ACOs of variations in spending growth. N Engl J Med 2012;10:366.

62 Pollack C, Armstrong K. Accountable care organizations and health care disparities. J Am Med Assoc 2011;305:1706–7.

# CHAPTER 13

# The legal framework for hospital emergency care

## Sara Rosenbaum

Department of Health Policy, School of Public Health and Health
Services, The George Washington University, USA

## Introduction

Hospital emergency care offers one of the most potent examples of the
extent to which the law influences and shapes medical practice. The
unique body of law that applies to hospital emergency departments
(EDs) did not happen overnight; it is instead a reflection of the extent to
which law is shaped by social experience over time.[1] Two strains fed this
fundamental shift in social expectations toward hospital EDs. The first
is the major advances in emergency medicine itself that occurred over
the course of the twentieth century, transforming health care in medical
emergencies from merely valuable to invaluable. The second was the
emergence of hospitals, during the second half of the twentieth century, as
major financial and power centers that received substantial public support
while wielding heavy influence in their communities. By the end of the
century this combination of technological achievement and financial and
medical power had triggered a fundamental restructuring of the law,
which recasts hospital EDs as what the law terms public accommodations
with basic obligations to serve those in need of emergency medical care.
This obligation to serve the public is virtually unknown in other parts of
the private health care sector.

At the same time, this legal metamorphosis contains important limitations that circumscribe hospitals' obligations in times of medical
emergency. In the quarter century since the enactment of the Emergency
Medical Treatment and Labor Act (EMTALA), courts and federal agencies

*Emergency Care and The Public's Health*, First Edition.
Edited by Jesse M. Pines, Jameel Abualenain, James Scott and Robert Shesser.
© 2014 John Wiley & Sons, Ltd. Published 2014 by John Wiley & Sons, Ltd.

have refined the scope of the law in order to constrain its reach. In a handful of instances, Congress also has stepped in to modify its terms. Yet EMTALA has withstood the test of time – and has survived even the nation's most ambitious effort at universal insurance coverage – not only because of the many gaps that remain in the wake of passage of the Affordable Care Act (ACA), but also because EMTALA reflects not only law but also broader public expectations regarding the role of hospitals in society.

Laws as significant as EMTALA typically do not emerge in one mighty flash. Instead, the pathway to sweeping legislation such as EMTALA is more gradual and multigenerational. Indeed, in the case of EMTALA, the roots of the law can be found in early common law (i.e., judge-made law) decisions handed down by state courts that broke new ground regarding the relationship between hospitals and society.[2] Judicial rulings were followed by the passage of emergency hospital care laws in a number of state legislatures, usually as conditions placed on licensure. Only after this base was in place did Congress take the ultimate step of making access to care in times of medical emergency a condition imposed on virtually all Medicare-participating hospitals. In short, the story of EMTALA, like those of other landmark laws, is one of evolution over time, across bodies of law, and in multiple legal venues.

This chapter examines EMTALA in the broader context of legal evolution. It provides an overview of EMTALA's precursors, describes the law in some detail (along with its implementing regulations), and discusses key issues that have arisen in the law's implementation. This chapter focuses on EMTALA rather than on the entire body of federal, state, and local law that shapes emergency medicine; such an analysis would consume an textbook. Instead, what is examined here is the nation's only federal law that indisputably, and despite its limitations, creates a legal right of access to care.

## First principles – no right to healthcare and no corresponding duty of care

It is a tenet of the law that health care providers owe their patients a duty of reasonable care.[3] What constitutes reasonable care, how reasonable care is to be measured, and how far the obligation should extend (i.e., whether it applies to health care institutions as well as medical professionals) are key factors that have changed over time, as courts and legislative bodies alike have witnessed the emergence of a modern health care system.[4] But the principle that health care providers owe a duty of reasonable care to their patients is fundamental to the US legal system. Medical liability law is principally one of state law and, to a greater or lesser degree, the doctrine of medical liability exists in all states.[5]

But medical liability doctrine comes with a major caveat: liability can arise only when a provider–patient relationship has been established, since it is this relationship that gives rise to the duty of reasonable care. Of crucial importance, therefore, are the interlinked common law principles on which the reasonable care duty rested: first, there is no right to health care; and second, there is no corresponding duty to furnish health care, even in medical emergencies. Put another way, at common law, there was no duty of rescue.[6]

It is difficult to overstate the importance of these twin doctrines, which together permitted physicians (and, by extension, the hospitals to which they admitted their patients) to select the people they would treat. To the extent that hospitals offered emergency services, care was accessible only to patients of the medical staff; even where hospitals employed residents, physicians, and other health professionals in their EDs, the staff retained the discretion to select the patients they would treat.[7]

Over the years, state and federal laws modified the no duty principle to bar certain health care providers from using discriminatory criteria to select their patients. For example, the 1964 Civil Rights Act made it unlawful for federally assisted entities (including hospitals and physicians that are considered to receive federal financial assistance under the law) to deny care to otherwise eligible people (i.e., those who could pay for care) on the basis of race or national origin.[8] Even more far-reaching is the Americans with Disabilities Act (ADA), which classifies the services of private health care providers as public accommodations. Under this standard, hospitals, physicians, and other providers of health care are barred from discriminating against qualified persons with disabilities regardless of whether they receive federal funding.[9] State human rights statutes similarly may bar discrimination by health care providers against people who can pay for care on prohibited grounds such as race, national origin, disability, gender, or sexual orientation.

But a bar against discrimination on a narrow range of prohibited grounds is a far cry from a broad abrogation of the "no duty" principle. As important as they are, antidiscrimination laws do not bar health care providers from refusing to accept patients into their care on grounds such as an inability to pay for care, no personal physician, residence outside a particular community, Medicaid coverage, or some other nonprohibited basis unrelated to the need for care. In other words, although civil rights laws constrain health care providers from arbitrarily withholding treatment from protected classes of persons, they do not create an affirmative duty to furnish care to people who need it, regardless of economic, social, or cultural factors. The no duty of care principle is best illustrated by a 1901 case, which remains good law today, in which "for no reason whatsoever" a physician refused to come to the aid of a woman dying in labor, despite the fact that she previously had been his patient. She had no legal right to emergency treatment, and he bore no liability for her death since he had no duty to treat her.[5,10]

## Cracks in the wall

As hospitals' place in the social order evolved, so did the thinking of the courts and legislative bodies.

### Shifting common law doctrine

Beginning in the latter half of the twentieth century, judicial doctrine began to shift away from the no duty principle where access to emergency hospital care was concerned. Although these cases were handed down by state courts and thus were binding only in the states in which they were decided, the decisions set precedents for other courts to follow. In some instances, courts declined to extend these evolving common law doctrines to their states.[8] In other states, courts reached the same conclusion: that hospital care in times of medical emergency had simply become too important, and hospitals' position in society too central, to continue to grant providers such discretion over when and whether to furnish emergency care.

Probably the most important case in this regard was *Manlove v. Wilmington General Hospital*.[11] The *Manlove* case involved an infant, sick for days with fever and diarrhea, whose condition continued to degenerate and whose parents sought emergency care. Because it was a Wednesday, their pediatrician, who had been caring for the infant, was not available, and they naturally turned to Wilmington Hospital, where the baby had been born. Here the Supreme Court of Delaware picks up the story:

> [The parents] thought that at the hospital the child would receive the help and relief that he so desperately needed. They further assumed that the mere sight of a child so sick, together with their recitation of his aggravated discomfort, would suffice to prompt someone to give aid while there was still time. But this was not the case, for they failed to account for the formality of admission requirements. The parents appeared before the nurse at her admissions desk in the Emergency Ward. They related the story of their child's illness and their doctor's treatment, and showed the medicine that had been prescribed. They further stated the child seemed to be failing, and requested that someone help him. The nurse apparently recalled her regulations to the effect that patients will not be admitted unless they present an admission slip signed by their physician. The nurse asked if they had such an admission slip and found that they did not. She stated that she would call the doctor's office. She did not discovered that the doctors were not available, whereupon she stated to the parents: "You have

no admission slip signed by your doctor and our regulations do not permit us to treat your child under the circumstances, but you may come back to our Pediatric Clinic tomorrow and someone will look after your child at that time." At no time had the nurse gotten up from her chair at the desk. At no time did she personally check the child. At no time did she make any effort to call an intern or staff physician, despite the fact that there were no patients in the Emergency Ward. The parents, having been denied treatment for their child, returned to their home and called [the pediatrician] to make an appointment for that evening. However, they never kept their appointment, for at approximately three o'clock the same afternoon the child was found to be dead in his crib. Cause of death: bronchial pneumonia.

The parents' lawyer in the subsequent wrongful death action, aware of the no duty principle, attempted to characterize the nurse's conduct as medical negligence, in this case, an incompetent and superficial diagnosis that had failed to elicit evidence of an emergency. The hospital lawyers, equally well aware of the no duty rule, instead sought to characterize the staff conduct as "nonfeasance," that is a failure to undertake care, which however morally regrettable, did not amount to a legal violation, because at common law there was no duty of care, not even in emergency cases involving hospital EDs.

The court began what turned out to be a breakthrough decision by considering the hospital itself, noting that while Wilmington Hospital was a private corporation, it was established as one that was to be "open to the public" (the very essence of a private enterprise that nonetheless is considered a place of public accommodation, much like hotels, inns, bus lines and other private transport businesses, and movie theaters).[9,12] Furthermore, as the court noted, the hospital, as a nonprofit corporation, received considerable public support in the form of tax exemptions, which were given not to benefit a limited class, but the community at large. As such, the proper characterization of the hospital was as a private corporation that existed to provide a public service. As such, the hospital's duties could be framed in relation to the community as a whole, not simply the patients it accepted for treatment:

> [The] defendant's argument . . . begins with the proposition that there can be no liability for misfeasance without a duty of reasonable care, or for nonfeasance without a duty to act. This duty may arise by statute or common law. There being no allegation of statutory duty we must look to the common law. It is then argued that the applicable common law rule is "essentially identical with that governing the physician in his practice," namely, that he is under no legal duty to accept any person

for treatment, no matter how extreme the emergency and that no duty attaches to the physician until he has actually undertaken to administer treatment . . . Assuming, without deciding, that a private physician may refuse to aid or treat in emergency cases . . . such a similarity cannot be said to exist in respect to the defendant. The attempted analogy fails for the simple reason that the defendant's acceptance of direct tax benefits, together with financial subsidies from the State, has of necessity changed its characterization to that of a quasi public institution, thereby forfeiting to a measured extent the degree of privacy that it otherwise possessed. It is abundantly clear to me that a hospital of defendant's character should be required at all times to render reasonable needed aid in those instances where an emergency involving death or serious bodily impairment might reasonably be said to exist. Of course, liability based on failure to fulfill this requirement is not absolute. The test is reasonableness. . . What I have said is an indication of . . . good policy.

The *Manlove* decision became a touchstone of modern health law, one whose holding and reasoning was extended to other jurisdictions. Concepts of public function, community reliance, and community benefit guided the thinking of courts around the country. Viewing hospitals in a modern light, an increasing number of state courts came to understand that a seismic shift had occurred in these institutions' place in society and, furthermore, that even though they were private, hospitals incurred public obligations, at least where medical emergencies were concerned.

### State statutes

Following on the heels of this shifting common law doctrine were state statutes, typically as an element of hospital licensure law, that codified common law principles in the form of legislation. State laws varied but were written to spell out in advance and in some detail the classes of hospitals to which the duty applied, the scope of their emergency care duties (e.g., screening, stabilization, medical transfers) and what constituted a medical emergency (e.g., imminent risk of death only, or, as in *Manlove*, an imminent risk of serious injury to health). The courts once again entered the picture in these state law cases, often because licensure agencies charged with enforcing the law were ill-equipped to monitor ongoing compliance or even to take decisive action in the event that an alleged violation of the law was reported. Thus, in *Thompson v. Sun City Community Hospital*[13] the issue was whether under Arizona's hospital licensure law, a Phoenix hospital treating a boy for a life-threatening injury could transfer him in an unstable state to the public hospital. The answer, according to the Arizona Supreme Court, was that state law as written compelled licensed hospitals with EDs not only to accept medical emergencies into care but to stabilize them before effectuating a transfer, and that this obligation applied even in cases in which a public hospital might be located in the same community.

### Federal precursor policies: The Hill Burton Act and Treasury/IRS rulings applicable to nonprofit hospitals seeking tax-exempt status

Although it is common to think of EMTALA as the first federal policy incursion into emergency medical care, this is not in fact the case. Two important predecessors laid the groundwork for the 1986 law. These predecessors themselves built on the evolution of common law standards outlined above, as well as earlier state efforts to enter the field as a matter of hospital licensure. The degree to which EMTALA is embedded in decades of policy – indeed, an extension of it – should not be overlooked.

The Hospital Survey and Construction Act of 1946 (popularly known as the Hill Burton Act) was enacted in order to spur the nationwide development of hospitals following the end of World War II. One of the earliest and most significant federal grant-in-aid programs, Hill Burton allocated funds to states that accepted its conditions of participation in order to construct hospital facilities. Two basic conditions that attached to facilities built with funding under the Act were first, a time-limited obligation to provide a reasonable volume of uncompensated care and, second, a perpetual obligation to serve the entire community. Federal regulations promulgated in 1979, over 30 years after enactment, spelled out these obligations in greater detail. The 1979 regulations interpreted the community benefit obligation as requiring, among other things, provision of emergency care without regard to ability to pay at the time services were rendered.[14] Surviving a legal challenge from the American Hospital Association, the regulations remain in effect today but apply only to nonprofit and public hospitals, since Hill Burton funding was not available for the construction of for-profit facilities.

A second major federal precursor policy to EMTALA can be found in Treasury/Internal Revenue Service policies interpreting the conditions that apply to public and private nonprofit hospitals that seek federal tax-exempt status. A seminal revenue ruling issued by the agencies in 1969, which set the broad contours for the modern "community benefit" standard against which hospital compliance is measured,[15] identified provision of emergency care regardless of ability to pay as a major factor in measuring hospital conduct.[16] The Patient Protection and Affordable Care Act amplifies and broadens the 1969 community standard but does not displace it.[17] As a result, provision of emergency care as a community benefit – and therefore, the abrogation of the common law "no duty" principle – remains core evidence of tax-exempt practice. Since many state and local tax-exempt statutes mirror federal tax-exempt policies, the federal emergency care evidentiary standard presumably would carry over into state and local tax policy as well.

## EMTALA

Several basic considerations ultimately led to EMTALA's passage as part of the Consolidated Omnibus Budget Reconciliation Act of 1985.[17] The first was the growth of the for-profit hospital industry, whose for-profit status placed it beyond the reach of either Hill Burton or Treasury/IRS rulings. Yet virtually all for-profit hospitals participated in the Medicare program.

The second factor was the 1982 enactment of the inpatient prospective payment system (PPS). The PPS statute's enactment in turn triggered concerns that patients would be discharged in an unstable state ("sicker and quicker," the saying went) by hospitals that, under the new payment system, would be incentivized to capture the maximum return on fixed payments by discharging Medicare beneficiaries prematurely and in an unstable condition. Studies of hospital behavior in the wake of PPS appeared to confirm this expectation.[18]

A third factor was the continued stories of patient dumping, that is, of hospitals' refusal to provide any treatment in medical emergencies or else to send patients with confirmed medical emergencies away in unstable condition. Of particular note were stories of widespread dumping on public hospitals by other Medicare participating hospitals. A year before, in response to these practices, the Texas legislature had enacted its own version of an anti-patient dumping statute, a move seen by federal policymakers as particularly notable in light of the state's hospital politics and the strength of its hospital industry.

The Congressional response to these considerations was EMTALA, a measure passed in virtually identical form[20] in 1985 by a Republican controlled Senate and Democratically controlled House and included in the 1986 Budget Act signed by President Reagan. Unprecedented in detail and scope, EMTALA has been amended in only relatively modest ways since its enactment. The Affordable Care Act affirmed EMTALA's primacy as a basic building block of the health care system; not only was Congress clear regarding hospitals' continuing EMTALA obligations,[19] but in amending the Internal Revenue Code's tax-exempt hospital provisions as part of the Act, lawmakers specified EMTALA compliance as an explicit condition of tax-exempt status.[20]

## EMTALA's two basic obligations: Screening and stabilization/transfer

The obligations of Medicare hospitals with EDs are spelled out at length in the statute,[21] as are other elements of the law such as methods of enforcement,[22] EMTALA's interaction with state laws,[23] whistleblower protections,[24] and a bar against delaying examination or treatment in order to enquire about insurance coverage or payment status.[25] In addition, the statute contains extensive definitions whose purpose is to reduce ambiguities related to the extent of hospitals' duties.

The basic EMTALA obligations, which reflect the bodies of law, reviewed above, that preceded it, can be summarized as follows.

### Medical screening requirement

EMTALA's fundamental breakthrough is the requirement that hospitals that have "hospital emergency departments" undertake care; that is, the law abrogates the "no duty" principle at common law. The undertaking must commence in the case of "any individual" who "comes to the emergency department" and on whose behalf a request is made for "examination or treatment for a medical condition." The individual need not make the request himself, nor is it lawful for a hospital to rely on a cursory glance to determine whether an emergency condition exists: its staff must undertake care, since the decision as to whether an emergency medical condition exists can be made only through "an appropriate medical screening examination within the capabilities of the hospital's emergency department, including ancillary services routinely available to the emergency department."[26] Nor is the existence of a medical emergency left to the discretion of a hospital; furthermore, EMTALA defines the concept of "emergency medical condition" as one involving an immediate threat to health, rather than life. As a result, the condition need not be life-threatening to qualify as one that triggers a hospital's further EMTALA obligations. Under the law, an emergency medical condition is:

> (A) a medical condition manifesting itself by acute symptoms of suffi-
> cient severity (including severe pain) such that the absence of immedi-
> ate medical attention could reasonably be expected to result in (i) plac-
> ing the health of the individual (or with respect to a pregnant woman,
> the health of the woman or her unborn child) in serious jeopardy; (ii)
> serious impairment to bodily functions, or (iii) serious dysfunction of
> any bodily organ or part; or (B) with respect to a pregnant woman
> who is having contractions – (i) that there is inadequate time to effect
> a safe transfer to another hospital before delivery; or (ii) that trans-
> fer may pose a threat to the health or safety of the woman or unborn
> child.[27]

## Necessary stabilizing treatment or appropriate transfer

Separate and apart from the screening requirement (as discussed below, the courts are split on the question of whether stabilization obligations arise only if preceded by a screening examination within the hospital's ED), a hospital must furnish stabilization treatment to "any individual" who "comes to a hospital" and is determined by the hospital to have an emergency medical condition. Stabilization services must be provided "within the staff and facilities available at the hospital" (in other words, not only the resources available to the hospital ED).[28] The law defines "to stabilize" as "to provide such medical treatment of the condition as may be necessary to assure, within reasonable medical probability, that no material deterioration of the condition is likely to result from or occur during the transfer of the individual from a facility."[29] Both transfers to other facilities and discharges qualify as a "transfer."[30]

In lieu of stabilization, EMTALA permits hospitals to transfer unstable patients under two narrowly drawn conditions. The first condition is the transfer trigger. For the hospital to engage in a medically unstable transfer under any situation, either the individual or his representative must request a transfer after being informed of the hospital's legal obligations and the risks associated with transfer, or a physician certifies in writing that the medical benefits of transfer outweigh the risks.

The second condition is the transfer itself, which must be "appropriate."[31] An appropriate transfer is extensively spelled out under the law and imposes an extraordinary duty on the transferring hospital that involves demonstrating not only that the transfer is appropriate but that the hospital's own resources (including its on-call specialists) are either inadequate or unavailable to the patient. Four conditions apply:

(A) The transferring hospital provides the medical treatment within its capacity which minimizes the risks to the individual's health, and in the case of a pregnant woman in labor, the health of the unborn child; (B) . . . the receiving facility – (i) has available space and qualified personnel for the treatment of the individual; and (ii) has agreed to accept the transfer of the individual and to provide appropriate medical treatment; (C) . . . the transferring hospital sends to the receiving facility all medical records . . . available at the time of the transfer, including records related to the individual's emergency medical condition, observations of signs or symptoms, preliminary diagnosis, treatment provided, results of any tests and the informed written consent . . . [as specified under the law], and the name and address of any on-call physician . . . who has refused or failed to appear within a reasonable time to provide necessary stabilizing treatment; (D) . . . the transfer

is effected through qualified personnel and transportation equipment.
. . [including necessary life support]; and (E) meets [other conditions
imposed by the Secretary].

## Enforcing EMTALA

One of the most powerful aspects of EMTALA is that the law expressly
allows for enforcement either by the Secretary of Health and Human
Services (HHS) (through the use of civil money penalties against hospitals
and her power to exclude from Medicare certain physicians who engage in
prohibited practices), or by individuals who suffer harm as a direct result
of a hospital's violation of its obligations. (The Affordable Care Act's community benefit amendments also make compliance with EMTALA an
explicit condition of tax-exempt status, thereby giving the IRS oversight
jurisdiction as well.) Individuals who are able to prove their claim are
entitled to civil money damages available for personal injury under the
laws of the state in which the hospital is located; as a result, state laws that
limit damages for medical injuries apply to EMTALA claims.[32]

EMTALA is generally thought of as reaching hospitals, but in certain
instances the Secretary can pursue enforcement against individual physicians (including on-call physicians) in the form of either financial penalties
or (in "flagrant" cases)[33] exclusion from Medicare. The conduct that can
trigger direct action by the Secretary against a physician entails: (i) mis-
representation of the risks and benefits of patient transfers, or (ii) misrep-
resentation of an individual's medical condition.[37] However, individuals,
in their private enforcement actions, are permitted to sue only hospitals,
not physicians.[36]

## EMTALA's application to specialized hospitals

The law extends its obligations beyond the immediate ED and hospital
facilities of the hospital to which the individual initially comes. Under
EMTALA, a Medicare-participating hospital that has "specialized capabilities or facilities (such as burn units, shock-trauma units, neonatal
intensive care units [or other capabilities specified by the HHS Secretary]"
is prohibited from accepting an appropriate transfer if "the hospital has
the capacity to treat the individual."[34] In other words, even if the specialized hospital is not the originating facility, and even if the emergency was
not initially identified within its four walls, it must accept an appropriate
transfer – that is, the specialized referral hospital is obligated to undertake
care unless it can show that it lacks the capacity to do so. In effect, the law
bootstraps the EMTALA obligations beyond the four walls of community
hospitals by requiring that specialty hospitals accept transfers unless they
lack capacity.

## EMTALA's interaction with state liability law

EMTALA is expressly designed to override the common law no duty of care principle where hospital emergency treatment is concerned. At the same time, its purpose is not to replicate or federalize state medical liability which, as noted, arises once a provider–patient relationship is established. For this reason, EMTALA expressly does not override state law.[27] At the same time, of course, once the undertaking commences (i.e., the screening, stabilization/transfer activities begin) it is possible that the same set of facts could give rise to both an EMTALA claim and a medical liability claim. Sorting out when EMTALA applies and when the case is a more straightforward medical liability case has come to occupy many courts, since, as noted previously, hospitals are so eager to avoid the ultimate exposure and potentially significant federal sanctions that accompany an EMTALA claim. Similarly, HHS, as discussed below, has attempted to delineate when a particular set of facts gives rise to an EMTALA claim and when the issue presented raises questions more appropriate to state medical liability law.

The numerous cases that have attempted to wrestle with this conundrum can be summarized as follows. The courts recognize as EMTALA claims situations in which the facts show a complete failure to screen an individual who comes to the hospital seeking care,[35] or provision of a discriminatory examination (one that is less than what the hospital would ordinarily undertake),[36] or the failure to stabilize a medical emergency before discharge or transfer,[37] or the failure to provide a medically appropriate transfer.[38] However, where a claim involves facts that a court comes to view as illustrating a substandard or incompetent screening examination, the case will be treated as a state law medical liability claim and the federal EMTALA allegation will be dismissed.[39]

Even this basic rule of thumb is problematic, since it is possible for situations to arise in which the facts presented could be understood *either* as a failure on the part of emergency room staff to follow their established protocols with respect to a particular patient, *or* a failure to properly identify a patient's symptoms to begin with as a result of negligent treatment. The patient suffers injury in either case. But in the former situation, an EMTALA violation potentially exists, while in the latter, the staff failure amounts to medical negligence. In hundreds of EMTALA cases brought by individuals over the years, the courts have wrestled with this Talmudic problem of characterization.

## Key issues in implementation

Because EMTALA is such a complex and detailed statute, and because the consequences of EMTALA violations are serious, the law has become a

complex battleground in both the courts and the federal agencies, as plaintiffs have sought to enforce what they perceive as comprehensive rights,
and as the hospital industry has sought to restrain the scope and reach of
the law with respect to the initial health care undertaking as well as the
extent and duration of their duty of care. A few of the more high profile
disputes are reviewed below.

### What does it mean to "come to" a hospital ED?

Under the statute, a hospital's EMTALA duty of care is triggered when an
individual "comes to" a hospital ED and a request is made for an examination for a medical condition. Final federal regulations issued in 2003,[40]
following numerous lawsuits to clarify these terms offer clarifications of
both "comes to" and "emergency department." The regulations are elab-
orate in their classification schemes for both terms, in recognition of the
various ways in which individuals may come to a hospital and the various points to which they may come. For example, an individual may walk
in the door of a hospital ED or may be brought by city ambulance. An
individual may arrive at an outpatient hospital clinical site, whereupon an
emergency arises during the course of care.

In order to determine whether the site to which an individual has come
amounts to an emergency department, the regulations create the concept
of a "dedicated emergency department," since, of course, emergency
departments are the hospital service site on which the premise of the
law rests. A "dedicated emergency department" (with the unfortunate
acronym DED) means "any department or facility of the hospital, regardless of whether it is located on or off the main hospital campus, which
meets at least one" of the following criteria: (1) the site is licensed as an
emergency department; (2) the site is held out to the public as available
for emergency or urgent care without an appointment; or (3) during the
preceding calendar year, at least one-third of all conditions treated at
the site (as measured through patient sampling) involved "outpatient
visits for the treatment of emergency medical conditions on an urgent
basis" without a previously scheduled appointment.[41] The 2003 Preamble
stresses that what is key in terms of the third criterion is how the site
actually functions and the type of care that it actually furnishes over the
course of a year. Thus, outpatient labor and delivery units, psychiatric
units, and sites that treat unscheduled cases all may qualify as sites that
must respond as an emergency department would respond.[42]

The regulations also clarify that "comes to" does not necessarily entail
literally walking (or being brought) through the hospital's ED doors;
simply being on hospital property (e.g., a parking lot, a sidewalk) can
satisfy the "comes to" test in health care situations presenting potential

emergencies, such as labor and delivery as well as serious injuries and illnesses.[48] The key under the rules is whether the individual has appeared on the hospital's main campus as opposed to a satellite clinic.

Particularly complex is the situation in which an individual is transported by air or ground ambulance. Use of ambulances to steer (literally) desirable patients to facilities and undesirable ones away has long been a well-recognized strategy employed by hospitals to cherry-pick patients, and to this day, instances are reported in which ambulance transports simply bypass facilities that they know will turn their patients away.[21] For this reason, the relevance of regulating hospital behavior in relation to ambulance transport remains high. The 2003 rules establish a two-tier hierarchy that turns on both hospital ownership and hospitals' broader community-wide responsibilities to respond to non-hospital-owned ambulance transports.

Where the hospital owns and operates the ambulance, an individual is deemed to have come to the hospital ED even prior to arrival at the ED itself. The only exception in such a situation occurs when the ambulance is being "operated under communitywide emergency medical services (EMS) protocols that direct it" to transport the patient elsewhere and furthermore is operating under the direction of a physician not employed by the hospital.[43]

In the case of non-hospital-owned ambulances, hospitals can avoid triggering a "comes to" situation – even in cases in which ambulance personnel call ahead and report that they are coming – if they place themselves on formal "diversionary status," meaning that they lack the resources or personnel to care for any additional patients.[52] Even here, however, the regulations clarify a hospital's obligation to accept the transport if the ambulance ignores the hospital's diversionary status and proceeds to its ED.[52]

In sum, the rules attempt to balance hospitals' ability to control patient flow through ambulance ownership with their broader community-wide obligation to remain accessible to patients whose business they do not seek. This attempt to strike a balance reflects prior EMTALA case law, in which the courts permitted hospitals to avoid community responsiveness only in formal diversion cases.[44]

### Must hospitals provide stabilization care even in situations involving patients whose conditions make medical treatment futile?

One of the most wrenching situations that can arise for any hospitals involves cases in which a person presents an immediate medical emergency but also has an underlying condition that, on a longer term basis, renders medical treatment futile. This extreme type of situation arose in the landmark case, *In the Matter of 'Baby K'*[45] in which a court clarified hospitals obligation to furnish stabilization treatment even in situations in which a patient has an underlying condition that is conclusively fatal. *Baby K* involved an infant born with anencephaly (a fatal condition in which an infant forms without a major portion of its brain and scalp and never attains consciousness even though reflexive skills such as breathing may continue to function, at least for a while). Following the mother's refusal of the normal standard of care in tragic cases such as this (i.e., warmth and hydration until the infant dies), Baby K was attached to a respirator but eventually breathed on her own. Periodically, however, she would experience apnea and would cease breathing; at this point, the nursing home where she resided would rush her to the hospital for emergency resuscitation.

Concluding that the presence of an underlying medical condition for which treatment was futile was irrelevant to a hospital's EMTALA duty to respond to an immediate presenting medical emergency, the United States Court of Appeals for the Fourth Circuit clarified the extraordinary nature of the law's stabilization obligation. It is an obligation that, in the view of the court, survives any longer term decision about how to approach a particular case. The decision effectively reflects the powerful duty imposed on hospitals by EMTALA, a statement regarding the legal obligation of US hospitals to utilize their extraordinary life-saving measures without regard to the long-term prognosis of any particular patient. Not surprisingly, perhaps, a comparable legal dispute to that which arise in the case of Baby K has not arisen in the 20 years since the decision was handed down.

As might be imagined, *Baby K* provoked an enormous response among legal scholars and practitioners. Equally unsurprisingly perhaps, given the profound issues that inevitably would arise were policymakers to attempt to place limits on EMTALA's reach in extraordinary cases involving profound disability or conditions that make treatment futile, (such as the Terry Schiavo case which culminated with an unprecedented instance of Congressional intervention in 2005),[46] the law has never been amended to exempt hospitals from the screening and stabilization obligations under specific circumstances related to health, life, or disability. (It is worth noting, however, that legislation introduced in 2011, but never enacted, would have exempted religious hospitals from EMTALA obligations that involved the provision of an emergency abortion where the life of the mother is in danger.[47])

### Do hospitals' stabilization duties apply to inpatients?

A particularly contentious issue over the years, and one that both the courts and the Department of HHS have revisited on numerous occasions, involves EMTALA's application to inpatients.[48] As noted previously, the legislative history surrounding passage of EMTALA suggests that the law was a Congressional response not only to the denial of ED care to indigent people, but also to concerns over the potential for the Medicare PPS payment system to incentivize the premature discharge of unstable Medicare beneficiaries. In this regard, the text of the statute itself seems to bear out the multiple levels of concern that underlay enactment. Clause (a) the screening obligation, defines a hospital's duty in relation to its "emergency department." That is, the duty to furnish a screening examination arises in cases in which an individual comes to the ED. However, clause (b), the stabilization obligation, references the hospital in its entirety. The language of clause (b) describes hospitals' stabilization duties in relation to individuals who come to a hospital. In the context of clause (b), the "comes to" reference is to the hospital in its entirety, not just its ED.

The courts became badly split on this issue. Some appellate courts concluded that clauses (a) and (b) operate entirely independently of one another, and therefore, that the clause (b) stabilization obligation can arise across all hospital departments and does not depend on the existence of a previous screening examination in the hospital ED. Thus, for example, if a scheduled cesarean delivery goes horribly wrong in the delivery room, the hospital bears an EMTALA stabilization obligation, even though the emergency condition was disclosed in a patient care setting far away from the ED. Under this interpretation, the EMTALA stabilization obligation applied regardless of whether an individual was an inpatient or an outpatient, and regardless of whether the emergency arose in connection with an emergency examination. This interpretation also appeared consistent with EMTALA's extension to hospitals with specialized capabilities, who are required to accept patient transfers. The patient transfer acceptance rule is not confined to patients in the ED, and yet without application of EMTALA's protections to inpatients, specialty hospitals would have no duty to treat, and thus, no duty to accept a transfer.

Other appellate courts disagreed. Instead they focused on EMTALA's most well-known purpose, namely, stopping the denial of care to indigent patients who present at hospital EDs. Instead they interpreted clauses (a) and (b) as being inextricably linked, so that the stabilization obligation applied only to persons who had received ED screening exams, and even then, only while they were still in the ED. As soon as they were admitted, these courts reasoned, normal principles of medical liability ensued since they were now patients of the hospital; EMTALA's special duty to treat was no longer relevant. These courts did not consider the problems associated with losing EMTALA protections as an inpatient in specialty transfer situations.

In an effort to resolve the conflict, the 2003 regulations specified that the stabilization obligation ceases upon admission of a patient from the ED as an inpatient unless a patient can demonstrate that the admission was undertaken as a subterfuge, that is, with the intent of extinguishing the hospital's EMTALA stabilization obligations. The 2003 rule also eliminated EMTALA protections entirely for individuals whose inpatient status is the result of a scheduled admission not carried out through the ED.[49] Beyond narrowing the stabilization protection to inpatients admitted through the ED, the rule thus establishes a very high burden of proof for persons whose admission is through the ED but who are then discharged in an unstable condition. Proving a subterfuge is virtually impossible, given the level of intent to deprive an individual of his or her rights that must be shown.

In the post 2003 regulatory climate, most courts that have considered the question of whether EMTALA applies to inpatients admitted through the ED have adopted the regulatory position. At least one appellate court, however, that applied EMTALA hospital-wide prior to the 2003 regulation has expressly refused to recognize the 2003 standard, concluding that the rule is in direct conflict with the language of the statute itself. Furthermore, on two occasions, HHS itself sought public comment on the question of whether its 2003 rule should be modified, recognizing the problem created for inpatients whose unstable conditions compel a specialty hospital transfer but whose status as inpatients have cost them their EMTALA protections. Ultimately the agency decided to leave its 2003 rule untouched.

### What are the on-call specialist obligations of hospitals under EMTALA?

Perhaps the highest profile battle fought out in the 2003 rules involved the question of on-call specialists, that is, the extent of hospitals' obligations to maintain robust specialist coverage for their EDs. Hospitals favored a strong standard given the difficulties they reportedly faced in recruiting sufficient specialists to provide ED coverage. Specialists, on the other hand, objected intensely to the on-call requirements in place under federal guidelines prior to the issuance of the 2003 regulations. While the failure of a hospital to have on-call specialists is not itself actionable by private individuals, the absence of specialists obviously has the potential to trigger numerous EMTALA issues such as failure of stabilization care, inappropriate transfers, and discriminatory screening examinations that fail to adhere to established protocols that require specialist consultation as part of the examination itself. Separate from EMTALA, of course, the absence of on-call specialist may raise serious questions from a medical liability perspective, as well as from the perspective of Medicare's conditions of participation.

In what was viewed as a win for the specialty groups, the 2003 regulations substituted a far more relaxed standard for on-call specialists than previously had been used by HHS in its EMTALA enforcement oversight. Under the 2003 standard, a hospital need only maintain an on-call specialist standard that "best meets the need" of its patients who receive EMTALA-related services.[50] Subsequent agency action limited this seemingly unfettered provider discretion over on-call specialist policies, but the question of on-call specialists remains elusive. Furthermore, since the presence of on-call specialists is not explicitly actionable under EMTALA unless one refuses to respond to a request from a member of the ED, simply lacking a roster of specialists raises no direct EMTALA considerations. HHS emphasized that its aim was to give hospitals more flexibility to attempt to come up with approaches that could balance the needs of their ED staff against the preferences and capabilities of specialists themselves.

## Conclusions

EMTALA is a landmark in US health law. At the same time it is an outgrowth of a half century of prior laws. EMTALA did not appear like some entirely unannounced *deus ex machina*. Instead, it evolved from a combination of remarkable technology advances, the emergence of hospitals as heavily publicly financed economic powerhouses, and shifting expectations regarding the role of hospitals in society.

Part of the rationale for EMTALA – the plight of the uninsured – can be expected to abate somewhat with the advent of national health reform. But as an enormous body of literature demonstrates – much of it reflected in other chapters of this book – the factors that underlie reliance on EDs go well beyond the lack of health insurance. Certain populations will always face enormous access difficulties, even with health insurance, as a result of their place of residence, their personal characteristics, their health conditions and disabilities, and other factors unrelated to the need for immediate medical attention. Furthermore, the weaknesses of the health care system itself, in particular the lack of adequate primary care – as well as appropriately functioning ambulatory specialty care access in many communities – lead to the use of EDs.

Because the factors that contribute to ED usage are so complex, Congress did not disturb EMTALA, even as it enacted legislation that over time may help reduce reliance on EDs. Indeed, precisely the opposite is true: Congress included in the ACA provisions that if anything reiterate the important role played by hospital emergency services, through insurance reforms aimed at ensuring that health plans cover emergency medical treatment, even when out-of-network.

Reducing dependence on ED care represents a long-term goal of health reform. It is possible that system reforms that strengthen the availability and accessibility of ambulatory care in high-need communities eventually will achieve this goal. Until then, hospital emergency care stands as one of the great achievements of the US health care system, and EMTALA stands as the nation's most fundamental legal statement regarding equity in health care access.

## Notes and References

1 Holmes OW. (1881) The Common Law.
2 As with the UK legal system, US law rests on the common law. Common law rulings and principles continue to play a foundational role in US law, despite the fact that so much of the legal framework that governs Americans today is found in statutes and implementing regulations that abrogate (i.e., modify) judicial rulings.
3 See, e.g., *Slater v. Baker and Stapleton* (1767) 95 Eng. Rpts. 860. In order to recover damages against a physician an injured patient must show that in rendering care, a physician had violated "the usage and customs of surgeons," that is, the professional standard of care owed all patients.
4 See Rosenbaum S, Frankford D, et al. (2012) Law and the American Health Care System, 2nd ed. Foundation Press. For example, it was not until the 1960s that hospitals were recognized as medical care institutions in their own right that, independent of their staffs, incurred a legal duty of reasonable institutional care. See *Darling v. Charleston Community Memorial Hospital* (1965) 211 N.E. 2d 253 . *Darling* involved a hospital's failure to furnish post-treatment monitoring care to a child with a broken leg, a lapse that ultimately led to the loss of the leg to gangrene. The decision is considered a landmark in US law, recognizing that separate from their medical staff, hospitals are obligated to hire capable staff and train them, monitor their performance, and generally to protect the health and welfare of their patients.
5 Rosenbaum S,Frankford D, et al. (2012) Law and the American Health Care System, 2nd ed. Foundation Press. Hospital liability takes two forms: vicarious liability, which occurs when the negligence of a member of the hospital clinical staff is imputed to the institution itself; and institutional negligence, when the hospital fails a patient in ways that are directly the responsibility of the institution. Thus, for example, a hospital can be vicariously liable if an emergency room physician in its actual or apparent employ performs negligently. The hospital may be institutionally (i.e., directly) liable if it was aware of prior acts of negligence by the staff member and failed to take proper corrective action.
6 For a discussion of the common law on this point see, *DeShaney v. Winnebago County* (1989) 489 U.S. 1891.
7 *Campbell v. Mincey* (1975) 413 F. Supp. 16. A federal trial court in Mississippi declined to extend common law decisions from other states abrogating the "no duty" principle to a case in which a woman about to deliver her baby was turned away from emergency care in part because the hospital did not consider a woman in labor to constitute a medical emergency. In summarizing the facts of the case, the judge characterized her delivery as "normal in all respects except for the location." Many of the most significant common law and statutory cases involving medical emergencies have concerned women in labor.

8 Hospitals and health facilities transferred to Public Health Service; restriction on closing hospitals 42 U.S.C. §2001 et. seq. For example, a physician who participates in Medicaid is considered to receive federal financial assistance under federal civil rights guidelines. See, e.g., HHS Office for Civil Rights. (2006) Guidance to Guidance to Federal Financial Assistance Recipients Regarding Title VI Prohibition Against National Origin Discrimination Affecting Limited English Proficient Persons. Available at: http://www.hhs.gov/ocr/civilrights/resources/specialtopics/lep/hhslepguidancepdf.pdf (accessed 30 November 2013).

9 See *Bragdon v. Abbott* (1998) 524 U.S. 624, barring a dentist from refusing treatment to a person with asymptomatic HIV on account of her HIV status (which is considered disabling under the ADA). Many ADA cases involve health care providers, specifically hospitals, that have been sued by individuals, or investigated by the Justice Department, for failure to make reasonable modifications to accommodate qualified persons with disabilities or for refusing to serve them altogether. *Howe v. Hull* (1994) 874 F. Supp. 779.

10 *Hurley v. Eddingfield*, 59 N.E. 1058 (Ind., 1901).

11 53 Del. 339 (1961).

12 The Civil Rights Act of 1964 classifies these types of enterprises as public accommodations subject to law's sweeping nondiscrimination rules. However, health care providers, including both physicians and hospitals, were not treated as public accommodations unless they received federal financial assistance such as grants and contracts. Passage of Medicare and Medicaid in 1965 dramatically broadened the reach of the Civil Rights Act, although in legislative history (not as an amendment to the Civil Rights Act itself), an exception was drawn for physicians who agreed to treat Medicare beneficiaries. See generally, Smith DB. (2001) Health Care Divided: Race and Healing a Nation. University of Michigan Press, Ann Arbor. It was not until 2000 that federal guidance governing language access limited the physician exemption to physicians who do not accept assignment of Medicare benefits.

13 688 P. 2d 605 (Ariz. 1984).

14 Provision of Services. (1979) 42 C.F.R. §124.603(b). The Hill Burton regulation did not define the term "emergency," however.

15 Revenue Ruling 69-545 1969-2 C.B. 117. For a discussion of the evolution of the community benefit standard, see, Rosenbaum S, Margulies R. (2011) Tax-exempt hospitals and the Patient Protection and Affordable Care Act: implications for public health policy and practice. 126 Public Health Rep. 2, 283–6.

16 See Peregrine M. et al. An overview of the additional tax exempt requirements for nonprofit hospitals. http://www.healthlawyers.org/hlresources/PI/Documents/FINAL_v4%20ARTICLE%20-%20An%20Overview%20of%20the%20Additional%20Tax%20Exemption%20Requirements%20for%20Nonprofit%20Hospitals%20(M%20Fin.pdf (accessed 30 Novmber 2013).

17 Consolidated Omnibus Budget Reconciliation Act Of 1985. (1986) Pub. L. 99-272. The one critical difference was that the House bill created private enforcement rights, while the Senate measure would have made enforcement exclusively the purview of the federal government. The Senate receded to the House on this matter. See Conf. Agreement to Accompany H.R. 3128. To date, hundreds of private EMTALA enforcement actions have been filed. No definitive empirical study exists

that classifies these actions by type of claim or plaintiff win/loss rates, although an educated observation by this author, who has read virtually all EMTALA decisions issued by the federal courts since decisions began to be handed down, is that plaintiffs are more likely to lose on the merits. That being said, the mere filing of an EMTALA suit undoubtedly is cause for concern on the part of hospitals, because the potential community and social impact are so much greater than a simple malpractice action. In a malpractice claim, the allegation against a hospital is that it breached its duty of reasonable care, a serious claim to be sure. But an EMTALA claim essentially is an allegation that the hospital has failed in its most fundamental duties to the community it serves.

18 For a discussion of the factors underlying EMTALA's passage, see Rosenbaum S, et al. (2012) Case studies at Denver Health: "patient dumping" in the emergency department despite EMTALA, the law that banned it. 31 Health Affairs 8, 1749–56.

19 See e.g., Patient Protections. (2010) P.H.S.A. §2719A requiring insurers to cover EMTALA-defined hospital medical emergency treatment without prior authorization and regardless of network status; PPACA §1303(d) related to continued obligation of hospitals to furnish emergency care for conditions related to pregnancy and abortion.

20 Exemption from tax on corporations, certain trusts, etc. 26 U.S.C. §501(r)(4)(B).

21 Examination and treatment for emergency medical conditions and women in labor. (1985) 42 U.S.C. §1395dd.

22 Examination and treatment for emergency medical conditions and women in labor. (1985) 42 U.S.C. §1395dd(d).

23 Examination and treatment for emergency medical conditions and women in labor. (1985) 42 U.S.C. §1395dd(f).

24 Examination and treatment for emergency medical conditions and women in labor. (1985) 42 U.S.C. §1395dd(i).

25 Examination and treatment for emergency medical conditions and women in labor. (1985) 42 U.S.C. §1395dd(h).

26 Examination and treatment for emergency medical conditions and women in labor. (1985) 42 U.S.C. §1395dd(a).

27 Examination and treatment for emergency medical conditions and women in labor. (1985) 42 U.S.C. §1395dd(e)(1).

28 Examination and treatment for emergency medical conditions and women in labor. (1985) 42 U. S.C. §1395dd(b).

29 Examination and treatment for emergency medical conditions and women in labor. (1985) 42 U.S.C. §1395dd(e)(3)(A).

30 Examination and treatment for emergency medical conditions and women in labor. (1985) 42 U.S.C. §1395dd(4).

31 Examination and treatment for emergency medical conditions and women in labor. (1985) 42 U.S.C. §1395dd(c)(2).

32 Examination and treatment for emergency medical conditions and women in labor. (1985) 42 U.S.C. §1395dd(d)(2)(A).

33 Examination and treatment for emergency medical conditions and women in labor. (1985) 42 U.S.C. §1395dd(d)(1)(B).

34 Examination and treatment for emergency medical conditions and women in labor. (1985) 42 U.S.C. §1395dd(g)

35 See, e.g., *Lewellen v. Schneck Medical Center* 2007 WL 2363384. Prisoner brought to a hospital with potentially life-threatening injuries was effectively found to have received no screening at all.

36 See, *Power v. Arlington Hospital Asso.* (1994) 42 F. 3d 851 (failure to appropriately screen a patient in a situation in which the hospital failed to follow its own established protocols for examining a patient presenting with symptoms like those of the plaintiff, whose undiagnosed infection and sepsis led to the loss of limbs and vision).

37 See *In the Matter of Baby K* (1994) 16 F. 3d 590 (4th Cir., 1994), establishing the duty of a hospital to stabilize a patient with an emergency medical condition even in cases in which the patient has an underlying medical condition that makes long-term treatment futile.

38 See *Cherukuri v. Shalala*, 175 F. 3d 446 (6th Cir., 1999), finding a transfer of unstable patients medically appropriate since all conditions for transfer of patients in such a situation were satisfied.

39 See e.g., *Summers v. Baptist Medical Center Arkadelphia* (1996) 91 F. 3d 1132 (failure to identify a broken back during a screening examination not an EMTALA violation, since the evidence presented demonstrated not that the physician failed to follow the standard screening protocol for the symptoms presented but instead failed to properly identify the symptoms to begin with).

40 68 Fed. Reg. 174 (2003) 53222-53264.

41 Special responsibilities of Medicare hospitals in emergency cases. (2012) 42 C.F.R. §489.24(b).

42 68 Fed. Reg. 53 (2003) 229.

43 Special responsibilities of Medicare hospitals in emergency cases. (2012) 42 C.F.R. §489.24(b)(3).

44 *Arrington v. Wong* (2001) 237 F. 3d 1066.

45 16 F. 3d 590 (4th Cir., 1994).

46 The case, which attracted intense national attention, involved a dispute over whether food and nutrition could be withdrawn from a woman who had spent 15 years in a persistent vegetative state. See, Quill T. (2005) Terry Schiavo – A Tragedy Compounded. 352 N Engl. J Med. 1630–3.

47 See Protect Life Act. (2011) H.R. 358. Sponsored by Representative Joe Pitts and co-sponsored by 100 members of Congress. The legislation was the outgrowth of a spectacular Arizona case in which a Catholic hospital's emergency staff performed a life-saving abortion and the nun who headed the ethics committee that made the decision to proceed given the threat to the mother was excommunicated. See Tenety E. (2010) On faith: Arizona hospital no longer "Catholic" after abortion to save mother's life. Washington Post http://onfaith.washingtonpost.com/onfaith/undergod/2010/12/st_josephs_hospital_no_longer_catholic_after_abortion_to_save_mothers_life.html (accessed 30 November 2013).

48 Rosenbaum S, Frankford D, et al. (2012) Law and the American Health Care System, 2nd ed. Foundation Press.

49 Special responsibilities of Medicare hospitals in emergency cases. (2012) 42 C.F.R. §489.24(d)(2)(i).

50 Special responsibilities of Medicare hospitals in emergency cases. (2012) 42 C.F.R. §489.24(j).

# CHAPTER 14

# The future of emergency medicine

**Robert Shesser**

*Department of Emergency Medicine, The George Washington University, USA*

## Evolution of US health systems

Despite widespread acknowledgment of its flaws, the fee-for-service (FFS) system of payment has remained the prevalent payment system in the United States[1] for decades. FFS is also the cause of a major economic schism between hospitals and physicians. About two-thirds of US physicians are currently engaged in single-specialty practice, either solo or small group through professional corporations and most hospitals are organized as not-for-profit entities. However, despite having "not-for-profit" in their title, most hospitals focus on increasing revenues, market share, and are often very aggressive in their relationships with physicians and other hospitals in their community. Interhospital competition and competition between physicians and hospitals for outpatient technical fees has caused poor allocation of available capital by the system as a whole.[2,3] Hospitals attempt to enhance high-margin care and invest significant capital in new technology, even when there is evidence of only marginal additional benefit.

For most of the twentieth century, a uniquely American practice model has evolved in which physicians in both longitudinal primary care and consultative practices evaluated patients in a practice setting both physically and corporately separate from the hospital. Physicians entered the hospital to perform procedures and manage the care of their hospitalized patients. In the US model, procedural and primary care physicians who practice independently die courted by hospitals to direct their patients to use that hospital's services. The competition by hospitals for physician-directed patients has been so intense that federal laws (Stark) have been promulgated that prohibit hospitals for paying physicians for

*Emergency Care and The Public's Health*, First Edition.
Edited by Jesse M. Pines, Jameel Abualenain, James Scott and Robert Shesser.
© 2014 John Wiley & Sons, Ltd. Published 2014 by John Wiley & Sons, Ltd.

referrals.[4] Outside the United States, there has been a stricter practice boundary divide between the self-employed outpatient physicians and their hospital-employed inpatient colleagues, who often have a more rigid (and often lower) salary structure than their independent practice colleagues.

In the United States, as medical practice delivery and management in the FFS environment (billing, coding, managed care contracting, malpractice insurance purchase, staff management, and benefits) have become more complex, many physicians in smaller single-specialty practice arrangements have seen benefit in ceding some practice autonomy, resulting in the development of larger groupings of physicians in a bewildering variety of practice arrangements. Medicine in the United States currently seems to be at the cusp of experiencing a major restructuring in the existing physician practice paradigm.

## A brief history of emergency care

Emergency medicine (EM) as a unique specialty in the United States originated in the late 1960s and rapidly evolved into its current form. Its emergence was driven primarily by increasing patient utilization of hospital-based emergency departments (EDs). Emergency physicians rapidly codified the body of knowledge required for its practice, developed training programs, a board-certification process, and several new national professional societies. A key element in this evolution and growth was the FFS system itself, which provided hospital managers with the incentive to invest in a physical plant to attract patients with undifferentiated illnesses for unscheduled care.[5] The FFS system's professional–technical split provided ED professional groups with their own revenue streams, permitting them to have practices that were financially independent of the hospital. The "community practice model" then evolved under which a hospital would contract with groups of independent ED physicians to guarantee adequate physician staffing of the ED. Emergency physicians would then refer "unattached" patients needing admission or aftercare to independent practitioners on the hospital's medical staff (the Alexandria Plan).

A major difference between EM and its hospital-based cousins was the early evolution of large single-specialty hospital contracting organizations as depicted in the satirical *Rape of Emergency Medicine*.[5] These organizations contracted directly with hospitals for EM professional services, employed their own physicians, and provided the full scope of practice management services. These organizations have played a major, albeit controversial, role in EM practice. One large national professional organization, the American Academy of Emergency Medicine, has vigorously opposed the "corporate ownership of ED contracts" describing it as both illegal and not in the best interests of patient care.[6]

Alternatives to the "community practice model" abound including closed-staff multispecialty integrated system models such as the Mayo or Cleveland Clinics where a parent organization runs the hospital and employs all the physicians; a hospital-employed model, often used in safety net hospitals whose payer mix is insufficiently robust to support FFS practice; and other public models such as the Veterans Health Administration or military systems in which physicians are publically employed.

The pressure for physician organizations to become larger is currently accelerating,[7] spurred by the high capital and technical requirements of electronic medical records systems and employer and government demands to lower health care costs which will ultimately require abandonment, or at least major modification, of the FFS system. Initiatives within the Affordable Care Act (ACA) take a "carrot and stick approach" that adds complexity to medical practice. Hospitals can receive higher payments or have payments refused based on quality or outcome metrics.

As hospital care represents about half of all health care costs, most of today's financial penalties and public reporting requirements relating to the ED are aimed primarily at the hospital,[8] but many decisions that financially impact the hospital are made by physicians. Today's hospital industry is in turmoil as each independent hospital or hospital system is refining its vision of the future, determining strategic direction, and investing considerable resources toward achieving those goals. The pressure is increasing on weaker hospitals to close or merge, which during the past decade has led to about an 18% decrease in US hospitals.[9] Many hospitals are reviewing their physician strategy, which in many cases means employing physicians or establishing some type of physician organization to do so.[10] Hospitals everywhere will therefore likely be assuming greater financial risk for the professional practices of both their hospital-based and (currently) independent physicians of their medical staff.

The details will vary locally, but the trend is clear: the current predominance of independent, single-specialty physician practice will change and whatever physician strategy is adopted by a hospital will soon be applied to its emergency physicians. ED physicians are the deckhands on the hospital's ship and the hospital's strategic direction will trump the desire of its contract physicians to remain independent. So the question for EM becomes: how can we best prepare for the new practice configurations that we will be compelled to accept?

## Future practice and funding of emergency medicine

The ability to make a living as an ED physician in the current system is based on generating FFS income based on the volume and complexity of services provided to a series of individual patients. In this model, ED physicians generally earn more than primary care physicians, because although ED providers treat similar numbers of patients per hour as do primary care physicians, ED physicians treat a higher acuity patient mix and perform more procedures. In certain situations, hospital revenues augment FFS emergency practice revenues to keep ED physicians' salaries high in less desirable geographic regions where board-certified ED physicians have been in short supply. ED physicians do not fund office-related expenses, which in most settings more than compensates for the higher malpractice and uncompensated care costs of EM practice. A shift away from a FFS model will change the basic economic foundation upon which EM has been built.

In order to continue attracting talented physicians to EM, salaries and working conditions will have to compare favorably with those of other specialties to justify ED physicians working a high proportion of off-hour and holiday shifts. Although marketplace factors of supply and demand cannot be ignored, there will be tremendous incentives for hospitals to create "managerial model" EDs where a relatively smaller number of emergency physicians (compared with today's "standard" staffing ratios) supervise the work of mid-level practitioners.

In the future, the number of ED physician jobs nationwide will be determined by aggregate ED patient volume, provider productivity, and any additional novel clinical and administrative positions staffed by emergency physicians within a redesigned health system. The supply will be determined by the number of residency graduates and the rate of retirement/specialty retention of those graduates. In addition to supply–demand issues, the relative compensation of ED physicians will be related to clinical productivity and the perceived value of these services.

## ED volume predictions

For decades, the worldwide health policy establishment has decried the use of the ED for minor illness.[11-14] The ACA will ensure that a greater proportion of the population has insurance and the number of nonhospital alternatives for patients with lower acuity illnesses will continue to increase. Therefore, EDs may experience a drop in the volume and proportion of lower acuity encounters. The degree to which the loss will be offset by increases in patients with chronic illness presenting for symptom exacerbations that require a rapid, intensive evaluation is unknown. The prevalence of chronic illness in our population should increase as there will continue to be more advances in palliative rather than curative treatments. ED visits from people becoming ill while traveling and health-seeking behavior by the uninsured, patients with psychiatric illnesses, substance abuse, and other complex social pathologies will likely continue at or below today's levels. Overall, it would seem reasonable to predict a general increase in the complexity of ED patients with a gradual decrease in rate of ED utilization in the United States. There will be a wide variation in the way different communities and health systems deal with the lower acuity after-hours unanticipated health needs. In some communities, treatment for these conditions may continue to center around EDs. In other communities, the continued development of retail clinics, urgent care centers, and extended hours with walk-in appointments in longitudinal care venues will significantly decrease a community hospital's ED census.

## ED staffing and provider mix

The specific stress points between the hospital and the ED medical group will change. Currently, hospitals pressure their FFS ED physician groups to provide more coverage. This pressure may be resisted by a group that wishes to minimize staffing costs and maximize provider take-home pay. In the future (as well as in present employed situations), ED physicians will be pressing the hospital for more coverage. This pressure may be resisted by a hospital that holds the professional practice financial risk. It is likely that with better governance, more precise quantitative ED management tools, and shared financial incentives, the ideal and most efficient mix between ED physicians, mid-level providers, and other physician aids (such as scribes) will be determined.

New measures will be developed to facilitate ED management and performance benchmarking:

1 *More precise measurement of ED case-mix acuity.* The current Emergency Severity Index (ESI) triage scale used in the United States is too imprecise for the acuity quantification of the ED patient stream, particularly because category III is so broad.[15,16] In addition, ESI is the prevalent triage tool, and many EDs still use time-based triage systems (i.e., how long patients can wait before seeing a physician), where there is poor inter-rater reliability. Accurately capturing acuity and case-mix will be necessary to explain differences among EDs. One potential approach would be to have two scales: one that could be applied on presentation and another that could be applied after evaluation and disposition that incorporated the intensity of the evaluations and their outcomes (e.g., admission percentage to various units, rapidity of outpatient follow-up required).

2 *Physician performance.* Many new measures will be developed as software is developed that can aggregate and normalize individual physician performance data. Productivity will be measured by patients treated per hour adjusted for the presence of mid-level practitioners and case-mix index. Throughput measures will focus on the intervals between when a patient is placed in a room and when a disposition decision is made similar to current systems. Measurements of admissions to general medicine and cardiology

(adjusted for the number of hours worked) where emergency physicians' judgment is generally exercised in a more unencumbered manner than in certain specialty area like psychiatry and surgical subspecialties will be tracked. Physicians may be measured on the intensity of cross-sectional imaging (studies per 100 outpatients seen), admission rates (admissions per 100 patients seen), laboratory utilization (tests per 100 outpatients seen), acute pain management (morphine equivalents administered in the ED per 100 patients treated) and outpatient narcotic utilization.

## ED practice boundary changes

The diffusion of technology (exemplified by the explosion of ED physician-performed ultrasonography) will continue. Modifications to the current FFS environment may establish a new ED sonography paradigm where it is in the interest of both the hospital and the radiologist to encourage a greater use of this modality in the ED. Accordingly, images will be routinely acquired in the ED by hospital-employed radiology technicians and interpreted by sonography credentialed ED physicians. Images may or may not be individually "over-read" by the radiologist, because they will be focused on answering a specific real-time clinical question rather than generating a bill. Archiving systems that store images, which can be easily linked to the patient's ED record, could also be developed.

New diagnostic modalities like the "pill-cam" will be used for the detection of gastrointestinal bleeding, and measurement of other gastrointestinal physiologic parameters which will provide new diagnostic insights. The days of nasogastric aspiration as a diagnostic test for upper gastrointestinal bleeding may soon end.

Noninvasive cross-sectional diagnostic imaging will continue to advance in speed and accuracy, expanding the armamentarium of ways to view three-dimensional structures, blood flow, and other dynamic metabolic processes. As advances in imaging will be the largest cost driver for an ED visit, there will be an explosion of rules to provide the clinician with guidance about which patients require emergent imaging. As major changes in the medical malpractice system are unlikely, the current dichotomy between physicians who attempt to practice strict evidence-based medicine and those who take a more liberal approach to diagnostic imaging and admissions will continue. However, a more robust physician's "report card" will provide health system managers with detailed feedback about a physician's resource utilization relative to their peers. It is safe to assume that increased pressure will be placed on high utilizers to bring their ordering practices and admitting practices into the group's normal range.

Continued evolution of information systems may effect a material change on the way ED visits are conceptualized by both patients and providers, on the way resident are trained, and on how the "value" of each visit is measured. Future information technology (IT) systems will permit ED physicians to gain a rapid clear picture of the patient's complete history, and will facilitate the optimal sequencing and timing of post-ED care. ED physicians may be able to view all of the prior inpatient and outpatient records within their health system and user-friendly links to other regional health systems' records and regional databases (such as the narcotic registries) will further facilitate care. The ED visit will be less a snapshot and more integrated into the patient's continuum of care. The ED physician group will be more integrated into a hospital's (health system's) extended group practice, and treatment algorithms will be developed in a multidisciplinary fashion to manage patients' problem-specific diagnostic trajectories more efficiently. If a patient who is scheduled to receive a vaccination or a routine monitoring test happens to find themselves in the ED for an unanticipated injury, the IT system will remind the ED physician about what intervention is scheduled and the ED physician may order its performance during the ED visit, saving a primary care office visit and enhancing the overall "value" of the ED visit.

### ED physicians' role in health systems

The health system of the future will be much more proactive in managing its patients' care-seeking behavior than are today's distributed systems. A good model for the future is the type of command centers that have been developed to manage the Kaiser Permanente patients' after-hours needs.[17] Future iterations of these centers will provide a broader range of services and will need on-site physician direction. It is to be hoped that this direction will come from EM, as emergency physicians have an ideal skill for managing such centers. These centers will receive enquiries directly from patients via telephone or web conference, receive enquiries from long-term care facilities about resident's status changes, receive input from home-care workers/home health aides, and provide online medical guidance for prehospital care providers (see below). In addition to visual assessment, these centers may be able to receive a variety of information from remote physiologic monitoring sensors and a variety of new smart phone applications that will guide treatment interventions. Documentation of any intervention will flow seamlessly into the patient's health record. Information from multiple sources will be correlated, treatment decisions made, and resources will be dispatched to the patient's location whether in a hospice, long-term care facility, or hotel.

## Future of pre-hospital emergency medical service systems

The current public safety organizational paradigm of prehospital emergency medical service (EMS) must change because maximal value and optimal management of these important resources can only occur if EMS really becomes an integral part of a redesigned health system. Effecting this change in urban areas will require cooperation among the various large institutional providers of health care because EMS system design must have a community-wide prospective.[18]

The advantages of moving EMS from safety to health are many, but the major reasons include the following:

1 For years municipal fire departments have been accused of usurping EMS resources for non-EMS purposes. Without the confusion of dual mission of both fighting fires and providing pre-hospital EMS, the actual funding requirement for each of these vital services will become more apparent to both municipal administrators and the voting public. The funding streams for each can then be individually articulated and benchmarked.

2 The training and capability of the EMS workforce and the mobility afforded by installed transport and communication capabilities are grossly inefficient when they *only* support emergency stabilization and transportation services. The potential to provide a variety of home-based monitoring and intervention services has been long-recognized by EMS leaders, but innovation has been stifled by the rigid limitations placed on EMS providers in the public safety model.

3 Emergency medical technician burnout is increased when their jobs are limited to pre-hospital and/or emergency transport interventions. Hours of training and years of experience are lost when providers have no career pathway that would permit them to employ their skills in a variety of less rigorous hospital or outpatient settings. Imagine a cadre of ED technicians culled from the ranks of experienced pre-hospital providers.

4 Close medical coordination will be necessary to maximize the value of pre-hospital care. This will require interoperability between electronic medical records used by EMS and those used by the health systems with which they relate. This goal can best be achieved through organizational structure change.

In large urban areas it is likely that there will be large integrated health systems. In these situations, the health systems may need to develop a public utility corporation to provide emergency ambulance services that are available to the whole community, but will have enhanced functionality that could support a variety of outreach initiatives for each large health system. Other candidates for participating in the management of public utility regional EMS systems would include home care agencies, community hospices, homeless outreach programs, and detoxification centers.

## Emergency medicine workforce development

Residency training programs will continue their evolution from yesterday's "guild" model to today's structured adult education experiences designed with solid input from professional educators. EM will eventually adopt one training model, which will most likely be the PGY 1-3 experience (25% less expensive without objective long-term benefit to society) with a robust series of Accreditation Council for Graduate Medical Education supervised fellowships to produce needed subspecialists. Programs may be encouraged to reduce systemic training costs through content sharing arrangements, made possible by development and distribution of digital educational content through the web.

Mid-level practitioners will continue their trend toward specialization and will continue to push organized medicine and public licensing agencies to gain more independence than they are currently afforded in most jurisdictions. The schism between physician assistants (PAs) and nurse practitioners will likely continue, though PAs may rebrand themselves to drop the word "assistant" from their title and create a new name for their expanded role.

The ED scribe role will continue to evolve as physicians working in the ED will need some sort of clerical administrative support to maximize their efficiency. The current scribe model could evolve while electronic health record systems' interoperability are improving into a "data miner" role which optimizes the bidirectional information flow through multiple patient databases.

## Conclusions

EM leaders today must prepare for new practice organization, practice boundaries, and the evolution of new roles within large health systems for emergency physicians. Their main focus must be to continually increase the value of each patient encounter by proper timing and sequencing of diagnostic testing, development of protocols with primary and specialty care colleagues, and working to lower barriers for bidirectional information flow. Increased efficiency in ED workforce development can be achieved through similar educational interspecialty and intraspecialty collaborations using web-based technologies.

## References

1 Mayes R. Moving (realistically) from volume-based to value-based health care payment in the USA: starting with medicare payment policy. J Health Serv Res Policy. 2011;16(4):249–51.

2  Thompson E. Duking it out: local hospitals fight back as physicians bring on competition with specialty facilities. Mod Healthc. 2000;30(29):3, 6, 9.

3  Lynk WJ, Longley CS. The effect of physician-owned surgicenters on hospital outpatient surgery. Health Aff (Millwood). 2002;21(4):215–21.

4  Payton B. Physician–hospital relationships: from historical failures to successful "new kids on the block". J Med Pract Manage. 2012;27(6):359–64.

5  Phoenix T. The Rape of Emergency Medicine. Cambridge, MA: Phoenix Publishers, 1992.

6  American Academy of Emergency Medicine. AAEM History. Available at: http://www.aaem.org/about-aaem/aaem-history (accessed 1 December 2013).

7  Mechanic R, Zinner DE. Many large medical groups will need to acquire new skills and tools to be ready for payment reform. Health Aff (Millwood). 2012;31(9):1984–92.

8  Centers for Medicare and Medicaid Services. Hospital Quality Initiative. Available at: http://www.cms.gov/Medicare/Quality-Initiatives-Patient-Assessment-Instruments/HospitalQualityInits/index.html (accessed 1 December 2013).

9  Harrison JP, Ferguson ED. The crisis in United States hospital emergency services. Int J Health Care Qual Assur. 2011;24(6):471–83.

10  Sowers KW, Newman PR, Langdon JC. Evolution ofphysician-hospital alignment models: a case study of comanagment. Clin Orthop Rel Res. 2013;471(6):1818–23.

11  Redstone P, Vancura JL, Barry D, Kutner JS. Nonurgent use of the Emergency Department. J Ambul Care Manage. 2008;31(4):370–6.

12  Gentile S, Vignally P, Durand AC, Gainotti S, Sambuc R, Gerbeaux P. Nonurgent use of the emergency department: a French formula to prevent misuse. BMC Health Serv Res. 2010;10:66.

13  Sempere-Selva T, Peiró S, Sendra-Pina P, Martínez-Espín C, López-Aguilera I. Inappropriate use of an accident and emergency department: magnitude, associated factors, and reasons – an approach with explicit criteria. Ann Emerg Med. 2001;37(6):568–79.

14  Pereira S, Oliveira e Silva A, Quintas M, Almeida J, Marujo C, Pizarro M, et al. Appropriateness of emergency department visits in a Portuguese University hospital. Ann Emerg Med. 2001;37(6):580–6.

15  Grossmann FF, Zumbrunn T, Frauchiger A, Delport K, Bingisser R, Nickel CH. At risk of undertriage? Testing the performance and accuracy of the emergency severity index in older emergency department patients. Ann Emerg Med. 2012;60(3):317–25.e3.

16  Platts-Mills TF, Travers D, Biese K, McCall B, Kizer S, LaMantia M, et al. Accuracy of the Emergency Severity Index triage instrument for identifying elder emergency department patients receiving an immediate life-saving intervention. Acad Emerg Med. 2010;17(3):238–43.

17  Berniker KJ. Life at EPRP: The Emergency Prospective Review Program. Perm J. 2001;5:4.

18  Delbridge TR. EMS … agenda for the future. Emerg Med Clin North Am. 2002;20(4):739–57.

# Index

AAPA. *see* American Academy of
    Physician Assistants (AAPA)
ACA. *see* Affordable Care Act (ACA)
access block
    in Australia, 23–4
accountable care organizations
    (ACOs), 154
    in payment reform, 154–6
Accreditation Council for Graduate
    Medical Education, 199
ACEM. *see* Australasian College for
    Emergency Medicine (ACEM)
ACEP. *see* American College of
    Emergency Physicians (ACEP)
ACOs. *see* accountable care
    organizations (ACOs)
active learning
    in improving patient outcomes, 89
acute care
    telemedicine in, 75–86. *see also*
        telemedicine
ADA. *see* Americans with Disabilities
    Act (ADA)
Advance Payment Model, 154, 155
Affordable Care Act (ACA), 7, 9, 12,
    84, 154, 159, 170, 176, 193
    ED utilization effects of, 102–3
Agency for Healthcare Research and
    Quality, 15, 51, 92, 157
aging
    emergency care in Singapore and,
        38–9

American Academy of Emergency
    Medicine, 192–3
American Academy of Pediatrics, 154
American Academy of Physician
    Assistants (AAPA), 103
American College of Emergency
    Physicians (ACEP), 18, 116
    2003 survey by, 17
American Heart Association
    HeartCode ACLS program of, 90
American Medical Association
    PCPI of, 159
American Recovery and Reinvestment
    Act (ARRA), 67, 84
American Well, 81
Americans with Disabilities Act
    (ADA), 171
anthrax dissemination incidents, 114,
    120, 127
Arizona Supreme Court, 174–5
ARRA. *see* American Recovery and
    Reinvestment Act (ARRA)
assumption of risk
    in payment reform, 162
Australasian College for Emergency
    Medicine (ACEM), 22–3
Australia
    access block and crowding in,
        23–4
    emergency care in, 22–4
    hospital and system capacity in, 24
    Kids Kare Line in, 80

*Emergency Care and The Public's Health*, First Edition.
Edited by Jesse M. Pines, Jameel Abualenain, James Scott and Robert Shesser.
© 2014 John Wiley & Sons, Ltd. Published 2014 by John Wiley & Sons, Ltd.

Bar Coding Management
  Systems, 53
BigPharma, 82
biosurveillance
  defined, 131*b*
bundled payments
  in payment reform, 157–8
Bureau of Labor Statistics, 103

Canada
  ED utilization in, 25
  emergency care in, 24–7, 26*t*
  emergency physician training in,
    25–6
  issues in emergency medicine in,
    26–7, 26*t*
Canada Health Act, 24
capitation models
  in payment reform, 153
cardiopulmonary resuscitation (CPR)
  Rescusci Annie in, 90
care coordination
  within communities, 144–5
  current literature on, 143
  defined, 142
  ED in, 8–9, 141–9
  within EDs, 143–4
  within hospitals, 144
  importance of, 141–3
  introduction, 141
  levels of, 141
  measurement of, 142
  problems related to, 146–7
care delivery systems
  ACOs, 154–6
  in payment reform, 154–7
  PCMH, 156–7
CDC. *see* Centers for Disease Control
    and Prevention (CDC)
CDR. *see* cognitive dispositions to
    respond (CDR)
CDSS. *see* clinical decision support
    systems (CDSS)
CEMP. *see* Comprehensive Emergency
    Management Program (CEMP)
Centers for Disease Control and
    Prevention (CDC)
  in emergency and disaster
    response, 117

Risk Based Funding
    Program of, 124
Centers for Medicare and Medicaid
    Innovation (CMMI), 155, 159
Centers for Medicare and Medicaid
    Services (CMS), 15, 84, 154,
    159–60
  Meaningful Use Menu Set
    Measures of, 142–3
Civil Rights Act (1964), 171
Cleveland Clinic, 193
clinical decision-making
  in emergency care, 53–4
clinical decision support systems
    (CDSS), 54
Clinical Information System, 83
Club of Mainz, 116
CMMI. *see* Centers for Medicare and
    Medicaid Innovation (CMMI)
CMS. *see* Centers for Medicare and
    Medicaid Services (CMS)
CODC. *see* Communication and
    Operations Directing Centers
    (CODC)
cognitive dispositions to respond
    (CDR), 53
College of Family Physicians of
    Canada, 25
Committee on Aging Issues
  in Singapore, 38–9
common law doctrine
  shifting, 172–4
Communication and Operations
    Directing Centers (CODC), 34
communication errors
  medical-related, 88
community(ies)
  care coordination within, 144–5
Community Care of North
    Carolina, 157
Comprehensive Emergency
    Management Program
    (CEMP), 115
Comprehensive Planning Guide 101
  of FEMA, 136
computed tomography (CT)
  in ED, 4
computerized provider order entry
    (CPOE) systems, 52–3, 60, 65, 70

Consolidated Omnibus Budget
    Reconciliation Act of 1985, 176
continuity of care
    forms of, 142
contract(s)
    EDs with hospital, 16–17
CPOE systems. *see* computerized
    provider order entry (CPOE)
    systems
CPR. *see* cardiopulmonary
    resuscitation (CPR)
Crew Resource Management, 92
Crisis Resource Management, 92
CT. *see* computed tomography (CT)
CVS Caremark Corporation, 106
CVS MinuteClinic, 106
cyberchrondia, 81–2

day-to-day operations
    continuity of, 132
deliberate practice
    in improving patient
        outcomes, 89
demographic(s)
    EDs impacted by, 101–2
Denmark
    emergency care in, 27–9
Department of Health
    in United Kingdom, 40–1
Department of Health and Human
    Services (DHHS), 67, 119,
    121, 183
    Hospital Preparedness
        Program of, 114, 119
Department of Homeland
    Security, 118
Department of Veterans
    Affairs (VA), 117
DHHS. *see* Department of Health and
    Human Services (DHHS)
diagnosis
    errors of, 87
diagnosis related groups (DRGs), 152
Disaster Medical Assistance Teams
    (DMATs)
    of US National Disaster Medical
        System, 121
disaster medicine

relationship with medical and
    health emergency
    management, 117
Disaster Medicine Section
    of ACEP, 116
disaster preparedness
    simulation in, 93–4
disaster response, 111–38. *see also*
    emergency and disaster
    response
DMATs. *see* Disaster Medical
    Assistance Teams (DMATs)
DNP. *see* Doctor of Nursing Practice
    (DNP)
Doctor of Nursing Practice
    (DNP), 105
Domestic Preparedness Program
    (DPP), 114
DPP. *see* Domestic Preparedness
    Program (DPP)
DRGs. *see* diagnosis related groups
    (DRGs)

Early Warning Infectious Disease
    Surveillance program, 132
Eastern Main Medical Center (EMMC)
    teletrauma by, 78–9
ED. *see* emergency department(s) (ED)
"ED boarding," 11
EDIS. *see* emergency department
    information system (EDIS)
educational efficacy in health care
    evaluation of, 89
efficacy research, 89
EHCs. *see* emergency health care
    coalitions (EHCs)
EHRs. *see* electronic health records
    (EHRs)
electronic health records (EHRs)
    in emergency care, 52
    first generation ED, 6
    hindrance of ED performance
        by, 4
    history of, 59
    impact on ED workforce, 104
    in online consultations, 80–1
    in payment reform, 161–2
ELSTs. *see* emergency life-saving
    technicians (ELSTs)

emergency(ies)
public health functions during,
127–8
rapidly evolving, 120–1
"Emergency 115," 34
emergency and disaster response,
111–38
conceptual relationship between
"disaster medicine" and
"medical and health
emergency management"
in, 117
disaster medicine evolution to
broader discipline of medical
and health emergency
management in, 116–17
enhancement of public health and
health care services
continuity through
interrelationship of public
health and health care
services emergency
management in, 117–18
evolution of emergency concepts
and terminology in, 118–19
future of, 122–4
health care systems in, 113–16, 115f
HVA in, 114
interaction as part of broader
health care system in,
119–20, 120f
interface between public health
and emergency health care
delivery during rapidly
evolving emergencies in,
120–1
medical response teams in, 121–2
organizational management in, 117
past and present, 113–22, 115b, 120f
programs created for, 114–15
specialty health care services and
medical surge in, 118
emergency care. see also emergency
departments (EDs)
acute, 75–86. see also telemedicine
EHRs in, 52
future of, 10
history of, 192–3

hospital. see hospital emergency
care
human factors in, 6–7, 47–58. see
also human factors in
emergency care
international perspectives on, 5–6,
21–44. see also specific
countries and international
perspectives on emergency
care
IT in, 59–74. see also information
technology (IT)
legal issues in, 9–10
misconceptions about, 5, 11–20. see
also misconceptions about
emergency care
myths about, 5
new payment reform policies
effects on, 9, 154–60
payment reform in, 151–67. see also
payment reform
simulation in, 87–96. see also
simulation
technology in, 45–96
emergency care system. see also
emergency care
described, 3–10
introduction, 3–5
in US, 1–44
emergency care workforce, 99–109. see
also emergency department (ED)
workforce
emergency department(s) (ED). see
also emergency care
boundary changes in, 196–7
in care coordination, 8–9, 141–9.
see also care coordination
"come to," 181–2
contracts with hospital, 16–17
crowding in, 4
CT in, 4
described, 3
diagnostic technology in, 4
EHRs in, 4, 6
emergency medicine, 197
evolving technology in, 7
FACEM-led, 23
fragmentation of care in, 4
"frequent fliers" of, 13

inpatient admissions from, 3
medical errors in, 6–7
misconceptions about, 11–20. *see
    also* misconceptions about
    emergency care
in national preparedness, 8
rate of annual utilization of, 11
staffing and provider mix for,
    195–6
transformation of care in, 3
volume predictions for, 194–5
emergency department information
    system (EDIS), 48
COPE in, 60
described, 59–60
ED workflow supported by, 63–4
features of, 59–63, 60*f*–3*f*
hospital-integrated, 62
patient disposition in, 61, 61*f*
RFID in, 60
sharing EHRs by, 62–3
snapshot dashboard or operational
    summary of ED in, 61–2, 63*f*
support of admitted patients by,
    61, 62*f*
value of, 65
emergency department information
    system (EDIS) adoption, 65–7
barriers to, 65–7
emergency department (ED)
    measures, 15–16
emergency department (ED) provider
    access
telemedicine in, 79–80
emergency department (ED)
    scribes, 106
emergency department (ED) staffing
current models of, 104–6
emergency department (ED)
    utilization
ACA effects on, 102–3
rapid growth of, 99–101
emergency department (ED)
    workflow
EDIS supporting, 63–4
emergency department (ED)
    workforce, 99–109. *see also*
    emergency department (ED)
    utilization

current models of staffing in, 104–6
current numbers, 103–4
EHRs impact on, 104
future directions for, 7–8
misconceptions about, 11–20. *see
    also* misconceptions about
    emergency care
population growth and changing
    demographics effects on,
    101–2
potential future models of, 106–7
projections, 103–4
emergency health care
multi-faceted role of, 113–26
emergency health care coalitions
    (EHCs), 115, 123
emergency life-saving technicians
    (ELSTs)
in Japan, 35–6
Emergency Management Committee,
    115
"Emergency Management Plan," 115
emergency management preparedness
    planning, 115, 115*b*
emergency medical service(s)
    (EMS), 103
in France, 30–1
pre-hospital, 198
emergency medical service center
    (EMSC)
in Japan, 36
Emergency Medical Treatment and
    Active Labor Act (EMTALA), 9,
    100, 169–70
application to specialized
    hospitals, 179
described, 176
enforcing, 179
hospitals' stabilization duties
    application to inpatients,
    183–5
implementation issues, 180–1
interaction with state liability
    law, 180
in legal framework for hospital
    emergency care, 175–87
meaning of "come to" a hospital
    ED, 181–2

Emergency Medical Treatment and
Active Labor Act (EMTALA),
(*continued*)
medical screening requirement
of, 177
obligations of, 177–9
on-call specialist obligations of
hospitals under, 185–6
in situations making medical
treatment futile, 182–3
stabilization/transfer requirement,
178–9
emergency medicine
boundary changes in, 196–7
evolution of US health systems
in, 191–2
future of, 191–200
future practice and funding of,
193–7
payment reform and, 160–1
performance gaps in, 87–8
physicians' role in health
systems, 197
staffing and provider mix, 195–6
volume predictions, 194–5
emergency medicine workforce
development of, 199
emergency operations
continuity of, 132
Emergency Operations Plan (EOP),
115
emergency physician training
in Canada, 25–6
emergency preparedness, 111–38. *see
also* emergency and disaster
response
emergency public health, 123, 127–38
challenges facing, 132, 135
as defined discipline, 135–7
existing policies in, 131–2, 133*t*–4*t*
functions of, 129–31
introduction, 127
legislation and presidential
directives for, 133*t*–4*t*
requirements for, 127–8
emergency response, 111–38. *see also*
emergency and disaster
response

Emergency Services Collaborative
in United Kingdom, 40
Emergency Treatment and Active
Labor Act, 161
EMS. *see* emergency medical service(s)
(EMS)
EMSC. *see* emergency medical service
center (EMSC)
EMTALA. *see* Emergency Medical
Treatment and Labor Act
(EMTALA)
environmental assessment
simulation in, 93
EOP. *see* Emergency Operations Plan
(EOP)
episode bundles
in payment reform, 158–9
episode of care
example, 158
"ER Wait Times Strategy," 26
ergonomics
application to emergency care,
47–58. *see also* human factors
engineering (HFE)
errors in prevention, 88
errors in systems, 88
errors in treatment, 87
errors of diagnosis, 87
essential public health services, 128–9,
128*b*
evidence-based care
in payment reform, 162

FACEMs. *see* Fellows of Australasian
College for Emergency
Medicine (FACEMs)
FCC. *see* Federal Communications
Commission (FCC)
Federal Communications Commission
(FCC) Broadband Plan, 75, 76*f*
Federal Emergency Management
Agency (FEMA), 121
Comprehensive Planning Guide
101 of, 136
federal precursor policies
in legal framework for hospital
emergency care, 175–6
fee-for-service (FFS) model, 151, 191–3

Fellows of Australasian College for
  Emergency Medicine (FACEMs)
  of ACEM, 23
FEMA. *see* Federal Emergency
  Management Agency (FEMA)
FFS model. *see* fee-for-service (FFS)
  model
FIRESCOPE, 117
France
  ED crowding in, 31, 31*t*
  ED(s) in, 30
  emergency care in, 29–31, 31*t*
  EMS: "stabilize and go" in, 30–1
  heat wave of 2003 in, 31
  medical schools and emergency
    medicine in, 30
FRCP-EM
  in Canada, 25
"frequent fliers"
  of EDs, 13
frontline healthcare workers
  human factors in emergency care
    applied to, 54
funding
  of emergency medicine, 193–7

Geisinger Health System, 157, 159
George Washington University, 4

hazards vulnerability analysis (HVA)
  in emergency preparedness, 114
HCAHPS. *see* Hospital Consumer
  Assessment of Healthcare
  Providers and Systems Survey
  (HCAHPS)
HCRT. *see* Healthcare Coalition
  Response Team (HCRT)
health care
  educational efficacy in, 89
  multi-faceted role of,
    113–26
health care services emergency
  management
  relationship with public health,
    117–18
health care system(s)
  in emergency and disaster
    response, 113–16, 115*f*

interaction as part of broader,
    119–20, 120*f*
health information technology (HIT),
    67–71, 68*t*–71*t*
  components of, 67
  core and menu objectives, 70–1, 71*t*
  hospital clinical quality measures,
    70, 70*t*
  hospital core objectives, 68*t*, 69
  hospital menu set objectives, 69, 69*t*
  ONC for, 67
  Robert Wood Johnson Foundation
    report on adoption of, 65–7
Health Information Technology for
  Economic and Clinical Health
  (HITECH) provisions, 84
Health Insurance Portability and
  Accountability Act (HIPAA)
  compliance, 83
health IT
  in emergency care, 52–3
Health Resources and Services
  Administration (HRSA), 103
health systems
  evolution of, 191–2
Healthcare Coalition Response Team
  (HCRT), 119, 122
healthcare workers
  human factors in emergency care
    applied to, 54
HeartCode ACLS program
  of American Heart Association, 90
HEICS. *see* Hospital Emergency
  Incident Command System
  (HEICS)
HFE. *see* human factors engineering
  (HFE)
HHS. *see* Secretary of Health and
  Human Services (HHS)
HICS. *see* Hospital Incident Command
  System (HICS)
Hill Burton Act, 175, 176
HIPAA compliance. *see* Health
  Insurance Portability and
  Accountability Act (HIPAA)
  compliance
HIT. *see* health information
  technology (HIT)

HITECH provisions. *see* Health
Information Technology for
Economic and Clinical Health
(HITECH) provisions
HMICU. *see* Hospital Mobile and
Intensive Care Unit (HMICU)
H1N1 influenza pandemic of 2009, 127
hospital(s)
care coordination within, 144
on-call specialists obligations
under EMTALA, 185–6
specialized, 179
"Hospital-Based Emergency Care At
the Breaking Point," 11
Hospital Compare Outpatient Quality
Reporting initiatives, 15
Hospital Consumer Assessment of
Healthcare Providers and
Systems Survey (HCAHPS), 160
hospital emergency care
legal framework for, 169–90. *see
also* legal framework for
hospital emergency care
Hospital Emergency Incident
Command System (HEICS), 117
Hospital Incident Command System
(HICS), 117, 123
Hospital Mobile and Intensive Care
Unit (HMICU)
in France, 30–1
Hospital Preparedness Program
of DHHS, 114, 119
Hospital Readmissions Reduction
Program, 160
Hospital Survey and Construction Act
of 1946, 175–6
Hospital Value Based Purchasing
(HVBP), 160
HRSA. *see* Health Resources and
Services Administration
(HRSA)
human factor(s)
in EDs, 6–7
in medical errors, 88
human factors engineering (HFE)
application to emergency care,
47–58. *see also* human factors
in emergency care
described, 47

methods, 47–9
observational analysis in, 48
simulation in, 49
task analysis in, 48–9
human factors in emergency care,
47–58
application to frontline health care
workers, 54
clinical decision-making, 53–4
health IT, 52–3
HFE methods, 47–9
interruptions, 51–2
overcrowding, 50
teamwork, 50–1
workflow, 49–50
Hurricane Katrina, 115–18
Hurricane Sandy, 118
HVA. *see* hazards vulnerability
analysis (HVA)
HVBP. *see* Hospital Value Based
Purchasing (HVBP)

ICS. *see* Incident Command System
(ICS)
*In the Matter of 'Baby K,'* 183
Incident Command System (ICS), 117
Incident Command System
(ICS)/National Incident
Management System
(NIMS), 137
Incident Management Teams, 119
India
emergency care in, 32–3
information exchange
in payment reform, 161–2
information technology (IT)
EDIS features in, 59–63, 60*f*–3*f*. *see
also* emergency department
information system (EDIS)
EHR history in, 59
in emergency care, 59–74. *see also*
emergency department
information system (EDIS)
health, 52–3
informational continuity of care, 142
Institute of Medicine, 51
Intermountain Healthcare Medical
Group, 157

international emergency care, 5–6, 21–44
international field medical teams, 121
International Health Regulations, 135
international perspectives on emergency care, 21–44
Australia, 22–4
Canada, 24–7, 26*t*
Denmark, 27–9
France, 29–31, 31*t*
India, 32–3
introduction, 21–2
Iran, 33–5
Japan, 35–7
Singapore, 37–40, 38*f*, 39*f*
United Kingdom, 40–1
interpersonal continuity of care, 142
interruptions in emergency care, 51–2
Iran emergency care in, 33–5
Iran Medical University, 35
IT. *see* information technology (IT)
iTriage, 84

JAAM. *see* Japanese Association for Acute Medicine (JAAM)
Japan
ED visits in, 36–7
emergency care in, 35–7
hospital care in, 36
pre-hospital care in, 35–6
Japanese Association for Acute Medicine (JAAM), 36
JCAHO. *see* Joint Commission on Accreditation of Healthcare Organizations (JCAHO)
Joint Commission on Accreditation of Healthcare Organizations (JCAHO), 15, 88, 114

Kids Kare Line in Australia, 80

"La Machine," 90
leadership errors medical-related, 88
Lean, 49
learning

active, 89
mastery, 89
legal framework for hospital emergency care, 169–90
cracks in the wall, 172–6
federal precursor policies, 175–6
introduction, 169–70
no right to healthcare and no corresponding duty of care, 170–2
shifting common law doctrine, 172–4
state statutes, 174–5
legal issues in emergency care, 9–10
liability law
EMTALA's interaction with, 180
longitudinal continuity of care, 142

MACS. *see* Multiagency Coordination Systems (MACS)
*Manlove v. Wilmington General Hospital,* 172–4
mastery learning in improving patient outcomes, 89
Mathematica Policy Research, 157
Mayo Clinic, 82, 193
MCI. *see* Medical College of India (MCI)
Meaningful Use Menu Set Measures of CMS, 142–3
medical and health emergency management relationship with disaster medicine, 117
medical apps, 83–4
Medical College of India (MCI), 32–3
medical errors
causes of, 88
deaths due to, 87
in EDs, 6–7
medical liability doctrine, 171
medical liability law, 170–1
medical simulation. *see also* simulation
history of, 90–1
Medical Surge Capacity and Capability (MSCC) manual, 119, 120*f*
Medicare

Medicare (*continued*)
ACOs under, 154–5
PGDP of, 156–7
Medicare Shared Savings Program,
154–5
Medifund, 37
Medisave, 37–8
Medishield, 37
MedLine, 82
mHealth, 83
defined, 75
Ministry of Internal Affairs and
Communications
in Japan, 35
misconceptions about emergency care,
5, 11–20
care for most conditions treated in
ED is carefully measured and
reported to public, 15–16
clear-cut guidelines about which
ED patients should be
admitted to hospital, 14–15
ED frequent users have no
longitudinal care
relationships with other
doctors, 13
ED physicians are employed to
hospital and have practice
structure similar to other
physicians at hospital,
16–17
ED workforce consists of
physicians who failed to
succeed in "private practice,"
18–19
EDs inherently expensive relative
to alternative outpatient
settings for many visit
categories, 12–13
EDs used for "primary care," 11
"frequent fliers," 13
guidelines about what constitutes
"appropriate" ED use, 14
most ED patients are uninsured, 12
most US acute care hospitals have
proper staff and equipment
to care for all types of patient
problems, 17–18
mobile health

defined, 75
Model State Emergency Health
Powers Act (MSEHPA), 132, 135
MSEHPA. *see* Model State Emergency
Health Powers Act (MSEHPA)
Multiagency Coordination Systems
(MACS), 119

National Bioterrorism Preparedness
Program, 114
National Board of Health
in Denmark, 28, 29
National Disaster Medical System, 121
national emergency access target
(NEAT)
in Australia, 23
National Health Service (NHS)
of United Kingdom, 40–1
National Hospital Ambulatory
Medical Care Survey, 79
National Incident Management
System (NIMS), 118–19
National Institutes of Health Stroke
Scale (NIHSS), 78
national preparedness
EDs in, 8
National Quality Forum, 15
National Strategy for Biosurveillance,
131, 131*b*
naturalistic decision-making (NDM),
53
NDM. *see* naturalistic
decision-making (NDM)
NEAT. *see* national emergency access
target (NEAT)
*New York Times*, 82
NFPA 1600, 136
NHS. *see* National Health Service
(NHS)
NightHawk, 78
NIHSS. *see* National Institutes of
Health Stroke Scale (NIHSS)
NIMS. *see* National Incident
Management System (NIMS)
1986 Budget Act, 176
NPs. *see* nurse practitioners (NPs)
nurse(s)
projected growth of, 103–6
nurse advice lines

in telemedicine, 80
nurse practitioners (NPs)
    projected growth of, 105

observational analysis
    in emergency care, 48
OECD. *see* Organisation for Economic
        Co-operation and Development
        (OECD)
Office of the National Coordinator
        (ONC) for Health Information
        Technology, 67
Office of the US Capitol Attending
        Physician, 120
Office of US Foreign Disaster
        Assistance, 121
Oklahoma City bombing, 114, 121
Omnibus Budget Reconciliation Act of
        1989, 153
on-call specialists
    obligations of hospitals under
            EMTALA, 185–6
ONC. *see* Office of the National
        Coordinator (ONC)
online medical consultations
    in telemedicine, 80–1
operational medicine teams, 121
Organisation for Economic
        Co-operation and Development
        (OECD), 24
Original Fee-for-Service Medicare, 154
outcomes research, 89
overcrowding
    in emergency care, 50

PAs. *see* physician assistants (PAs)
Patient Access to Responsible Care
        Act of 1997, 153
patient-centered medical home
        (PCMH), 154
    in payment reform, 156–7
patient-centered triage tools
    in telemedicine, 81–2
Patient Choice System, 159
patient outcomes
    learning concepts related to, 88–9
Patient Protection and Affordable
        Care Act (ACA), 84, 175–6
pay for performance (P4P)

in payment reform, 159–60
payment reform, 151–67
    assumption of risk in, 162
    capitation models in, 153
    care delivery systems in, 154–7
    challenges facing, 161–3
    EHRs in, 161–2
    in emergency care, 151–67
    emergency medicine and, 160–1
    evidence-based care in, 162
    information exchange in, 161–2
    initiatives in, 152–4
    introduction, 151–2
    newer models, 9, 154–60
    physician payment initiatives in,
            157–60
    prospective payment system in, 152
    regional variations in care and, 163
    relative value scales in, 153–4
    vulnerable and high-risk
            populations and, 163
payment reform policies
    impact on emergency care, 9
PCMH. *see* patient-centered medical
        home (PCMH)
PCPI. *see* Physician Consortium for
        Performance Improvement
        (PCPI)
Pentagon crash site (2001), 121
performance gaps
    defined, 87
    in emergency medicine, 87–8
Pew Internet and American Life
        Project, 82
P4P. *see* pay for performance (P4P)
PGDP. *see* Physician Group Practice
        Demonstration (PGDP)
PHEP core capabilities. *see* Public
        Health Emergency
        Preparedness (PHEP) core
        capabilities
physician(s)
    future role in emergency medicine,
            197
physician assistants (PAs)
    projected growth of, 103–6
Physician Consortium for
        Performance Improvement
        (PCPI), 159

Physician Group Practice
  Demonstration (PGDP)
  of Medicare, 156–7
physician payment initiatives
  bundled payments, 157–8
  episode bundles, 158–9
  in payment reform, 157–60
  P4P, 159–60
  value-based purchasing, 159–60
Pioneer ACO Model, 154, 155
population growth
  EDs impacted by, 101–2
PPS. *see* prospective payment system
  (PPS)
pre-hospital emergency medical
  service systems
  future of, 198
preparedness activities
  in emergencies, 130–1, 131*b*
"prescription for fear," 82
prevention
  errors in, 88
primary stroke centers (PSCs), 77
Problem Oriented Medical
  Information Systems (PROMIS)
  at University of Vermont, 59
procedural skills training
  in simulation, 91–2
PROMIS. *see* Problem Oriented
  Medical Information Systems
  (PROMIS)
prospective payment system (PPS)
  inpatient, 176
  in payment reform, 152
ProvenCare, 159
PSCs. *see* primary stroke centers
  (PSCs)
public health
  basic functions of, 128–9, 128*b*
  emergency, 127–38. *see also*
    emergency public health
  relationship with health care
    services emergency
    management, 117–18
public health continuity of operations
  in emergencies, 128
Public Health Emergency
  Preparedness (PHEP) core
  capabilities, 130

public health preparedness
  defined, 127
public health recovery
  in emergencies, 128
public health services
  essential, 128–9, 128*b*
public health surge capacity
  in emergencies, 128

radio-frequency identification (RFID)
  technology, 60
*Rape of Emergency Medicine,* 192
RBRVS. *see* resource-based relative
  value scales (RBRVS)
REACH. *see* Remote Evaluation of
  Acute Ischemic Stroke (REACH)
relative value scales
  in payment reform, 153–4
  resource-based, 153–4
Remote Evaluation of Acute Ischemic
  Stroke (REACH), 77
remote patient monitoring
  defined, 75
  telemedicine in, 82–3
research
  efficacy, 89
  outcomes, 89
resource-based relative value scales
  (RBRVS), 153
response activities
  in emergencies, 130
Resusci Annie rescue-breathing
  simulator, 90
RFDS. *see* Royal Flying Doctor Service
  (RFDS)
RFID technology. *see* radio-frequency
  identification (RFID) technology
"right sizing"
  in ED staffing, 104
Risk Based Funding Program
  of CDC, 124
Robert Wood Johnson Foundation
  report
  on HIT adoption, 65–7
Royal Flying Doctor Service
  (RFDS), 23

SAMU, 30
SARS outbreak of 2003, 127

SBTT. *see* simulation-based team training (SBTT)
screening
  by EMTALA, 177
Second Life, 91
Secretary of Health and Human Services (HHS)
  in EMTALA enforcement, 179
September 11, 2001 terrorist airplane attacks, 114, 121
SGR. *see* sustainable growth rate (SGR)
simulation
  in disaster preparedness, 93–4
  in emergency care, 49, 87–96
  in environmental assessment, 93
  history of, 90–1
  improving care through, 91
  introduction, 87
  procedural skills training for, 91–2
  teamwork training for, 92–3
simulation-based team training (SBTT), 93
Singapore
  emergency care in, 37–40, 38*f*, 39*f*
  health care financing in, 37–8
  silver tsunami in, 38–9
  toward integrated care in, 39–40
Six Sigma, 49
SMRT. *see* specialized medical response team (SMRT)
SMUR, 30
Society and Chapter of Emergency Medicine of Singapore, 40
specialized hospitals
  EMTALA's application to, 179
specialized medical response team (SMRT), 121
stabilization
  by EMTALA, 178
"stabilize and go," 30–1
state liability law
  EMTALA's interaction with, 180
State Public Health, 119
state statutes
  in legal framework for hospital emergency care, 174–5
store and forward technology
  defined, 75
Supreme Court of Delaware, 172–4

sustainable growth rate (SGR), 153–4
system(s)
  errors in, 88

task analysis
  in emergency care, 48–9
teamwork
  in emergency care, 50–1
Tehran University of Medical Sciences, 35
Teledoc, 81
telehealth, 7, 75–86. *see also* telemedicine
telemedicine
  in acute stroke management, 77–8
  case studies, 76–9
  defined, 75
  in extending ED provider access, 79–80
  integration with quality drivers, 84
  medical apps in, 83–4
  mHealth in, 75, 83
  nurse advice lines in, 80
  online medical consultations in, 80–1
  patient-centered triage tools in, 81–2
  in rapid interpretation of radiologic images, 78
  in remote patient monitoring and follow-up, 82–3
  in traumatic injury management, 78–9
  at UMMC, 76–7
TelEmergency, 76
TelEmergency pilot program
  at UMMC, 77
TelEmergency Program Professor, 76
teleradiology
  case study, 78
telestroke
  case study, 77–8
teletrauma
  case study, 78–9
"The State of Emergency Medicine in Singapore," 40
*The Waiting Room*, 5

*Thompson v. Sun City Community Hospital*, 174–5
Tokyo subway Sarin attack, 114, 118
transfer
    by EMTALA, 178–9
Transitions of Care Committee, 142
Treasury/IRS rulings
    applicable to nonprofit hospitals seeking tax-exempt status, 175–6
treatment
    errors in, 87
Trust for America's Health, 132

UMMC. *see* University of Mississippi Medical Center (UMMC)
United Kingdom
    emergency care in, 40–1
United States (US). *see also under* US
    emergency care system in, 1–44. *see also* emergency care; emergency care system
    HIT policy of, 67–71, 68*t*–71*t*. *see also* health information technology (HIT)
United States (US) Court of Appeals for the Fourth Circuit, 183
University of Florida anesthesia portfolio, 90–1
University of Mississippi Medical Center (UMMC)
    telemedicine at, 76–7
University of Pittsburgh Medical Center, 81
University of Texas Health Science Center

    in Houston, 82–3
University of Vermont
    PROMIS at, 59
Urban Search and Rescue (US&R) task force, 121
US emergency and disaster response, 113–26. *see also* emergency and disaster response
US National Disaster Medical System
    DMATs of, 121
US&R task force. *see* Urban Search and Rescue (US&R) task force

VA. *see* Department of Veterans Affairs (VA)
value-purchasing based
    in payment reform, 159–60

WebMD, 82
workflow
    defined, 49
    ED, 63–4
    in emergency care, 49–50
workforce
    ED. *see* emergency department (ED) workforce
    emergency medicine. *see* emergency medicine workforce
workforce projections
    emergency care, 99–109. *see also* emergency department (ED) workforce
World Association for Disaster and Emergency Medicine, 116